Review Questions for
ULTRASOUND

A Sonographer's Exam Guide

Review Questions for
ULTRASOUND

A Sonographer's Exam Guide

by

Joyce A. Miller, Ed D, RDMS

Clinical Assistant Professor and Acting Chairman, Diagnostic Medical Imaging Program

Linda M. Chase, BA, BS, RDMS

Assistant Professor

Adrian C. Anthony, BS, RDMS, RDCS

Assistant Professor, Diagnostic Medical Imaging Program

Steven M. Ostrow, MD

Assistant Professor and Director of Undergraduate Education, Department of Radiology

State University of New York Health Science Center at Brooklyn

Review Questions Series
Series Editor: Thomas R. Gest, PhD
University of Arkansas for Medical Sciences

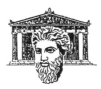

The Parthenon Publishing Group Inc.
International Publishers in Medicine, Science & Technology

One Blue Hill Plaza, Pearl River, New York 10965, USA

Published in the USA by
The Parthenon Publishing Group Inc.
One Blue Hill Plaza,
PO Box 1564, Pearl River,
New York 10965, USA

Published in Europe by
The Parthenon Publishing Group Limited
Casterton Hall, Carnforth,
Lancs LA6 2LA, UK

Library of Congress Cataloging-in-Publication Data

Review questions for ultrasound : a sonographer's exam guide / by Joyce A. Miller ...
[et al.].
      p.   cm. -- (Review questions series)
   ISBN: 1-85070-704-9
   1. Diagnosis, Ultrasonic -- Examinations, questions, etc.
I. Miller, Joyce A. II. Series.
   [DNLM: 1. Abdomen -- ultrasonography -- examination questions.
2. Ultrasonography, Prenatal -- examination questions. 3. Genital
Diseases, Female -- ultrasonography -- examination questions.   WI 18.2
R454 1998]
RC78.7.U4R48 1997
616.07'543'076 -- DC21
DNLM/DLC
for Library of Congress   97-42674
                                            CIP

British Library Cataloguing in Publication Data

Review questions for ultrasound : a sonographer's exam guide. - (Review questions
series)
   1. Ultrasonic imaging - Examinations, questions, etc.
   I. Miller, Joyce A. II. Sonography
   616'.07543'076

   ISBN 1-85070-704-9

This edition published 1998

Printed by J.W. Arrowsmith Ltd., Bristol, UK

PREFACE

This book contains review questions covering the areas of the abdomen and small parts, and obstetric and gynecologic ultrasonography, as well as a section devoted to the physics of ultrasound. The questions are provided with answers that also contain in-depth annotations and information, all of which have been developed to present students with the types of questions that are often asked in the examinations for these specialties. The audience targeted by this text includes:

♦ Sonographers or physicians who are preparing to take the Registry examinations administered by the American Registry of Diagnostic Medical Sonographers;

♦ Sonographers or physicians in the field who wish to assess and update their current knowledge; and

♦ Educators in ultrasound who wish to use this text to update their knowledge and/or develop test items.

Each section of this text is in the format of multiple-choice questions that are similar to those of the Registry examinations. Most answers, whether correct or incorrect, are explained and clarified. It is strongly recommended that these questions be used as a guide for establishing the areas in which the user needs additional review, which should then be obtained by referring to textbooks and articles on the subject.

**Joyce A. Miller, Linda M. Chase,
Adrian C. Anthony and Steven M. Ostrow**
Brooklyn

DEDICATIONS

This book is dedicated to our mentor and teacher, Dr. Mimi C. Berman, with sincere gratitude for her guidance, inspiration and friendship throughout the years, and:

— To my husband Michael, and our children and grandchildren Ahuva, Donny and Dvora, and Avrohom, Sora Malka and Adina; and to my parents Marty and Phyllis Feinstein, and my in-laws Anne and Philip Miller, with much appreciation for their love and support.

Joyce

— To my children Matthew, David and Sharyn, with love and appreciation for the inspiration, support and encouragement they have always given me; and to my grandchildren Sima, Akiva and Yeshaya, for the wonder they bring to everything.

Linda

— To my mom Claudia Alethea Browne, with sincere appreciation for all her words of encouragement and support, to whom I also wish a happy retirement in her new island home.

Adrian

— To the memory of Lucy Frank Squire, MD, who inspired me to become a radiology educator, and who demonstrated daily the value of using humor constructively in education and the importance of learning from one's students. For all this I am grateful.

Steven

GENERAL TEST-TAKING TIPS

Before the examination

The most important first step in successful test-taking is to BE PREPARED! You will do your best on any examination if you know the material. This means that you should prepare for the examination in a timely and organized manner. Schedule your study time so that you have an adequate amount of time for each section of material to be learned. Ideally, your study schedule will allow you enough time to review all the material at least one day before the examination and should avoid the need for a last-minute 'all-nighter'.

The next important preparation is to get a good night's sleep. Try to arrive at the examination venue a little early so that you can orient yourself and, if possible, choose a comfortable seat. Dress comfortably – you may need a sweater – and, by all means, use the facilities BEFORE entering the examination room.

Make sure you know what you are required to bring to the examination (i.e., your I.D., pencils, etc.) and have them ready in advance. Familiarize yourself with all policies and procedures relating to the examination.

Taking the examination

Unless otherwise directed, answer ALL of the questions. Scoring is based on the number of correct answers. There is no penalty for incorrect answers.

Pace yourself. Do not work so fast that you become careless, and do not spend a lot of time on questions that are too difficult. Use the 'best-guess' method to fill in an answer on your answer sheet, and mark the question in your test booklet. Time permitting, you can return to it at the end.

Always pay special attention to the instructions given before the examination and in the test paper. They are there to help you complete the examination correctly and efficiently. Time spent understanding the directions will save you time while taking the examination.

Read each question carefully and entirely, evaluating ALL choices before you decide which are the best. Then, eliminate as many wrong anwers as you can. It is easier to decide between two choices than among five. Make educated guesses, but do not 'second-guess' the question. Make sure that you are answering the question being asked, and not the one you think is being asked.

When you change an answer, make sure you have a good reason to do so; do not change answers on a last-minute 'hunch'.

If you are taking a paper-and-pencil examination, do not make stray marks on your answer sheet; make sure that your answers are clear and unequivocal. If you change an answer, erase the incorrect selection completely. If you are taking the test on computer, make sure that you understand how to operate the program.

CONTENTS

SECTION 3: OBSTETRICS AND GYNECOLOGY   **101**

SECTION 1: PHYSICS

Each section contains 200 questions in true/false and multiple-choice formats.

Elementary principles

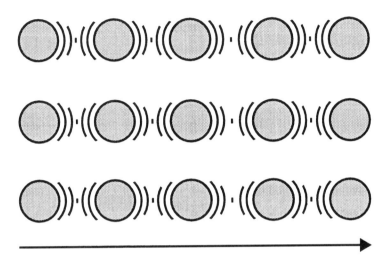

Use the above diagram to answer question 1.001.

1.001 The oscillation of particles occurs in a transverse direction relative to the beam width.
- A. true
- B. false

A is correct.
Ultrasound waves are considered longitudinal waves. This means that the oscillation of particles is in the direction of the propagation of the ultrasound energy. Therefore, both the direction of ultrasound energy propagation and the oscillation of the particles are perpendicular to the crystal face.

1.002 The effect of ultrasound on the medium results in particle motion which produces electrical, rather than mechanical, energy.
- A. true
- B. false

B is correct.
The piezoelectric principle describes the conversion of energy in the crystal from electric to mechanical (movement) energy. This mechanical energy is now transferred into the body.

1.003 With the velocity being constant, if frequency is doubled, wavelength is_____.
- A. increased by a factor of 2
- B. decreased by a factor of 2
- C. doubled
- D. none of above

A is correct.
The velocity of sound in soft tissue is 1.54 mm/μs. In ultrasound physics, it is considered a constant since wavelength × frequency = velocity. Thus, if one is increased, the other is decreased by the same magnitude; for example, if frequency is halved, then the wavelength is doubled.

1.004 If power (or gain), expressed as 40 dB, is reduced by 50%, the new gain is:
A. 20 dB
B. 60 dB
C. 37 dB
D. 80 dB

C is correct.
The decibel system was developed to allow comparison of two quantities. However, the difference between some quantities is so vast that a different scale has to be used. This scale is called the logarithmic scale. In decibel notation, the change in power by 50% is a 3-dB change; thus, the correct answer is 37.

1.005 With a 2-MHz transducer, in soft tissue, the wavelength is approximately:
A. 0.5 mm
B. 0.5 cm
C. 0.77 mm
D. 2.0 mm

C is correct.
The propagation speed is equal to the wavelength × frequency; thus, 1.54 mm/μs ÷ 2,000,000 cycles/s = 0.77 mm.

1.006 The energy per unit area of a sound beam is called:
A. power
B. amplitude
C. intensity
D. sensitivity

C is correct.
Power is the energy of the ultrasound beam and intensity is power divided by an area.

1.007 The peak pressure or height of a wave is known as:
A. A-mode
B. temporal average intensity
C. amplitude
D. frequency

C is correct.
Ultrasound has wave properties that are often displayed by a wave schematic. The wave schematic is also a scale that can demonstrate the change in acoustic variables. These changes in variable magnitude are also called changes in amplitude.

1.008 If density is increased, with everything else remaining the same, propagation velocity will:
A. increase
B. remain the same
C. decrease
D. none of the above

C is correct.
The propagation velocity is dependent upon medium density and elasticity. The more elastic the medium, the higher the propagation speed. Also, the greater the medium density, the lower the propagation speed.

1.009 If elasticity is increased, propagation velocity will:
A. increase
B. remain the same
C. decrease
D. none of the above

A is correct.
The propagation velocity is dependent upon medium density and elasticity. The more elastic the medium, the higher the propagation speed. Also, the greater the medium density, the lower the propagation speed.

1.010 The velocity of sound in a medium:
    A. decreases as compressibility increases
    B. is essentially constant with frequency changes
    C. dictates the wavelength if the frequency changes
    D. increases as elasticity increases
    E. all of the above

E is correct.

The velocity of sound in the medium is dependent upon the properties of the medium, particularly its elasticity and density. The sound propagation speed (velocity) increases with increasing elasticity, thereby decreasing compressibility and decreasing density. The frequency of the ultrasound is dependent upon the sound source. The frequency will remain the same regardless of the medium's characteristics. However, the wavelength will change according to the relationship between the frequency and the propagation speed of sound in that medium.

1.011 The letters 'SPTA' are a means of expressing:
    A. decibels
    B. pressure
    C. intensity
    D. amplitude

C is correct.

SPTA stands for 'spatial peak, temporal average'. This and other such designations describe conditions in which ultrasound intensity can be measured. 'Spatial peak' refers to the place in space where the intensity of the beam is at its highest. 'Temporal average' refers to the intensity of the beam, including both its transmit time and receive time.

1.012 In a 1-cm^2 area where the intensity is 7 W/cm^2:
    A. the power is 7 W/cm^2.
    B. the power is 7 W
    C. the power is 5000 mW/cm^2.

B is correct.

Power is defined as the rate of doing work. Intensity is defined as power over an area. If an intensity of 7 W is spread over 1 cm^2, then the intensity is 7 W/cm^2.

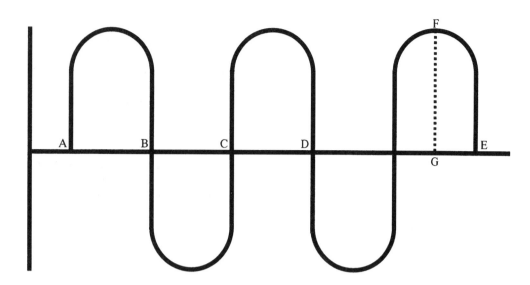

Use the above diagram to answer questions 1.013—1.016.

1.013 The interval A to B can be the :
  A. period
  B. wavelength
  C. none of the above

C is correct.

1.014 The interval C to E can be the:
  A. period
  B. wavelength
  C. both of the above

B is correct.

1.015 The interval A to E can be the:
  A. period
  B. wavelength
  C. spatial pulse length

C is correct.

1.016 F to G represents the:
  A. pulse amplitude
  B. pulse intensity
  C. pulse width

A is correct.

Propagation of ultrasound through tissues

1.017 Propagation of a sound wave through a medium will cause oscillation of particles around a point of equilibrium.
  A. true
  B. false

A is correct.
Huygen's principle is the established method for describing sound propagation through a medium. According to Huygen's principle, when sound propagates through a medium, it causes a particle to oscillate about a point of equilibrium and affects the successive particles adjacent to it.

1.018 The acoustic impedance mismatch between air   and soft tissue will be:
  A. low
  B. high
  C. equal
  D. inconsequential

B is correct.
The impedance of soft tissue is approximately 1,630,000 rayls and the impedance of air is 400 rayls. This is such a vast difference that sound is reflected to a higher degree between soft tissue and air than between soft tissue and bone (7,800,000 rayls).

1.019 The spreading out of a beam as it diverges from a central axis is:
  A. refraction
  B. reflection
  C. diffraction
  D. deflection

C is correct.
This is the definition of diffraction. The term diffraction is also used to describe spreading of the ultrasound beam after passing through a small aperture.

1.020 If the intensity transmission coefficient is 0.74, the intensity reflection coefficient will be:
  A. 1.06
  B. 6.00
  C. 0.26
  D. 0.04
  E. 0.40

C is correct.
The equation to use for this problem is $1 - IRC = ITC$. The ITC and IRC must add up to the total energy, or 100% of the overall energy, or 1: $0.74 + 0.26 = 1.00$

1.021 Acoustic impedance is defined as the product of:
  A. the mismatch between two interfaces
  B. a change in velocity at oblique incidence
  C. speed of sound in tissue and density of the tissue
  D. wavelength and frequency

C is correct.
The unit for acoustic impedance is $1 \ kg/m^2/s$, or the product of the density and the propagation speed.

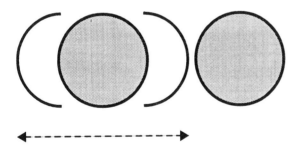

Use the above diagram to answer question 1.022.

1.022 The maximum displacement of a particle from its point of equilibrium, as sound propagates through a medium, is known as:
  A. refraction
  B. diffraction
  C. amplitude
  D. reflection

C is correct.
Particle displacement is one of the acoustic variables. The acoustic variables represent the amplitude changes that occur as sound passes through a medium.

1.023 Interfaces between media of greatly differing impedances are NOT a potential source of:
   A. amplitude
   B. attenuation
   C. artifact
   D. shadowing

A is correct.
Strong reflectors are usually associated with acoustic shadowing. Acoustic shadowing itself is an ultrasound artifact because it does not represent a true anatomic structure. The shadowing effect is caused by absorption, reflection or scattering of the ultrasound beam. These three are causes of ultrasound attenuation.

1.024 Which of the following correctly lists substances in an increasing order of ultrasound velocity?
   A. air, water, liver, bone
   B. bone, air, liver, water
   C. air, bone, water, liver
   D. bone, water, liver, air

A is correct.
In general, sound velocity increases with the increasing stiffness of the material. This rigidity in ultrasound is called elasticity.

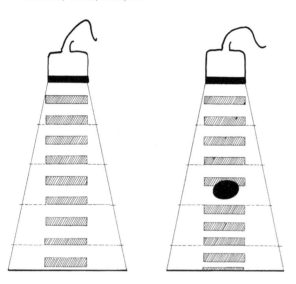

Use the above diagram to answer question 1.025.

1.025 A pulse of ultrasound travelling through soft tissue encounters a cystic structure. The pulse will then:
   A. speed up
   B. slow down
   C. maintain its initial velocity
   D. none of the above can be determined

B is correct.
The difference between soft tissue and a fluid-filled structure in ultrasound is: 1) the fluid-filled structure will attenuate the ultrasound beam less; and 2) the fluid is less rigid/elastic; therefore, the sound velocity through it will be less than through soft tissue. In this example, the pulse will slow down.

1.026 Rayleigh scattering is an example of:
   A. strong reflection
   B. specular reflection
   C. a reflector the same size or smaller than the wavelength
   D. side lobe artifact

C is correct.
This is the definition of Rayleigh scattering.

1.027 Refraction occurs when:
A. an interface is encountered at normal incidence
B. an acoustic impedance mismatch occurs
C. propagation velocities are equal
D. none of the above

D is correct.
Snell's law defines the relationship between the incident ray, the reflected ray, the transmitted ray, and their associated angles. For refraction to occur, the incident ray must strike the interface at an oblique angle and the propagation speeds of the two media must be different.

1.028 The most used diagnostic ultrasound range is:
A. 3.5–7.5 MHz
B. 2–10 MHz
C. 3.5–7.5 MHz
D. 3–20 MHz

B is correct.
The best answer is 2–10 MHz, as 10 MHz is used for some vascular work and 2–2.25 MHz for deep abdominal work.

1.029 Which of the following frequencies is NOT in the ultrasound range?
A. 10,000 Hz
B. 100,000 Hz
C. 1 MHz
D. 0.1 MHz
E. A and D only

A is correct.
The ultrasound range comprises frequencies > 20,000 Hz. In the choices listed, only 10,000 Hz is below 20,000 Hz. Note that 0.1 MHz is the same as 100,000 Hz.

1.030 To travel 1.54 cm in soft tissue, it takes a sound wave:
A. 1.54 seconds
B. 1.54 microseconds
C. 3.08 microseconds (roundtrip)
D. 10 microseconds

D is correct.
The speed of sound in soft tissue is 1.54 mm/μs or 1540 m/s. In the example, 1.54 cm is 10 times 1.54 mm. For the expression to be equal, microseconds (μs) must be multiplied by 10; therefore, the answer is 10 microseconds.

1.031 In soft tissue, if frequency is doubled, the half-value (intensity) layer will:
A. decrease by a factor of 2
B. double
C. remain the same
D. cannot be determined

A is correct.
The half-value layer is defined as the depth of a medium at which the ultrasound energy will reach half its starting or original value. Since the reduction in ultrasound energy is directly related to the attenuation, and the attenuation is directly related to the frequency of ultrasound used, the best answer is A.

1.032 As particles oscillate in a medium, attenuation occurs primarily through:
A. absorption
B. reflection
C. scattering
D. wavefront divergence

A is correct.
Attenuation is defined as the reduction of energy due to absorption, scattering and reflection. Reflection occurs at the level of the interface. Scattering is due to the dispersion characteristics of the medium. When particles move, they generate heat. The conversion of ultrasound energy to heat defines absorption.

1.033 Huygen's principle accounts for:
A. television imaging
B. superimposition of waves on a wavefront
C. time-gain compensation (TGC)
D. all of the above

B is correct.
Huygen's principle describes how each particle in the path of an ultrasound beam becomes a point source of sound. The wavelets that are generated are superimposed and become a planar wavefront.

1.034 The Schlieren system is a method of:
   A. predicting refraction angles
   B. determining the attenuation coefficient in bone or lung
   C. displaying a cross-section of the beam shape by employing acousto-optic interaction
   D. calculating the angle of far field divergence

C is correct.
To study the behavior of sound, a system has been devised to allow the beam to be seen. A technique that uses light called acoustic optical imaging has been developed. The Schlieren system is a well-known version of this technique.

1.035 If medium 2 impedance is equal to medium 1 impedance:
   A. 100% of the intensity will be reflected
   B. 100% of the intensity will be transmitted
   C. the reflection and transmission coefficients will be equal
   D. the answer cannot be determined without values given

B is correct.
An impedance mismatch is what causes ultrasound intensity to be reflected. If the impedances are the same and there is no impedance mismatch, there will be no reflection of energy and all of the energy will be transmitted.

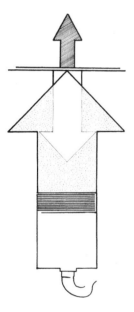

Use the above diagram to answer question 1.036.

1.036 At a bone–soft tissue interface:
   A. much more energy is transmitted than reflected
   B. much more energy is reflected than transmitted
   C. approximately as much energy is transmitted as reflected
   D. total internal reflection occurs

B is correct.
The impedance mismatch between bone and soft tissue is high and, therefore, most of the energy will be reflected.

1.037 A typical value of attenuation in soft tissue is:
   A. 0.1 dB/cm/MHz
   B. 1 dB/cm/MHz
   C. 19 dB/cm/MHz
   D. none of the above

B is correct.
The attenuation coefficient for soft tissue usually ranges from 0.5–1.1 dB/cm. This number assumes a 1-MHz frequency transducer. In this case, the best answer is 1 dB/cm/MHz.

1.038 When a sound wave encounters a soft tissue/soft tissue interface, approximately_____ % of the incident intensity is reflected.

 A. 1
 B. 15
 C. 25
 D. 50

A is correct.

For reflection to occur, the two media that the ultrasound traverses must have different impedances. Since all soft tissues have generally the same impedance, there will not be much reflection. In this case, the best answer is 1%.

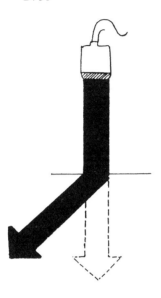

Use the above diagram to answer question 1.039.

1.039 A change in the direction of sound when crossing a tissue boundary is known as:

 A. diffraction
 B. refraction
 C. scattering
 D. wavefront

B is correct.

If sound traverses two media at an oblique angle and the propagation speeds of the two media are different, the path of the beam will be bent or changed. This phenomenon defines refraction.

1.040 The reflection of sound is greater in _____ than it is in _____.

 A. bone, air
 B. air, bone
 C. soft tissue, bone

B is correct.

The attenuation of sound in bone is high due to its high absorption coefficient and its high reflectivity. The attenuation in air is high due to its ability to scatter sound. When sound moves from soft tissue to air, there is greater reflection than in soft tissue to bone because there is a greater acoustic impedance mismatch.

1.041 The velocity of sound through bone is approximately:

 A. 408 cm/μs
 B. 15,400 cm/s
 C. 1.54 mm/μs
 D. 408,000 cm/s

D is correct.

The propagation speed of sound in a medium is determined primarily by its elasticity. Bone is much more rigid than soft tissue and produces a sound velocity of 4080 m/s.

1.042 The highest velocity occurs in which of the following?
   A. air
   B. bone
   C. tissue
   D. fat

B is correct.
Of the listed choices, bone has the highest elasticity and therefore the highest sound velocity.

1.043 Refraction at an interface may be caused by:
   A. velocities equal and a 30° angle of incidence
   B. velocities not equal and a 45° angle of incidence
   C. velocities equal and a 0° angle of incidence
   D. none of the above

B is correct.
Refraction occurs when a sound beam is incident upon an interface obliquely and the sound velocities of the two adjacent media are different.

1.044 Normally, at a specular reflector:
   A. the angle of incidence is equal to the angle of reflection
   B. the angle of incidence is 0°
   C. the angle of reflection is less than the angle of incidence
   D. the angle of transmission is equal to the angle of reflection

A is correct.
According to Snell's law, the angle of incidence is equal to the angle of reflection at a specular or smooth interface.

1.045 Sound travels through medium 1 and encounters an interface at an incident angle of 40°. The transmitted sound then enters medium 2 with a higher velocity.
   A. The reflected angle is 43° and the transmitted angle is 40°.
   B. The reflected angle is 40° and the transmitted angle is 43°.
   C. The reflected angle is 40° and the transmitted angle is 37°.
   D. The reflected angle is 37° and the transmitted angle is 43°.

B is correct.
If the angle of incidence equals the angle of reflection, then the reflected angle should be 40°. If sound passes from medium 1 to medium 2 obliquely and the two media have different propagation speeds, refraction should occur. If the sound velocity of medium 2 is greater than that of medium 1, the angle in that medium is expected to be higher. Thus, the best answer is a transmitted angle of 43°.

1.046 The reflection at the interface between water and air is approximately:
   A. 1%
   B. 25%
   C. 50%
   D. 100%
   E. 77%

D is correct.
The impedance difference between water and air is so high that most of the ultrasound energy will be reflected.

1.047 The reflection at the interface between fat and muscle is approximately:
   A. 1%
   B. 25%
   C. 50%
   D. 100%
   E. 77%

A is correct.
Fat and muscle have similar impedances. Most of the ultrasound will be transmitted.

1.048 Attenuation of 7 dB in 4 cm of tissue with an attenuation coefficient of 0.5 dB/cm will occur with a frequency of:
    A. 2.25 MHz
    B. 3.5 MHz
    C. 5.0 MHz
    D. 7.5 MHz

B is correct.
The attenuation of sound in tissue is determined by the attenuation coefficient of the tissue, the frequency of the sound, and the length or distance of the path that the sound has traveled. The equation is written: attenuation (dB) = attenuation coefficient (dB/cm) × frequency (cycles/s) × path length (cm). Therefore, 7 dB = 0.5 dB/cm × (unknown) × 4 cm. Rearranging the equation to solve for the unknown: (unknown) = 7 dB ÷ 0.5 dB/cm × 4 cm. The unknown is 3.5 and, therefore, the answer is 3.5 MHz.

Ultrasound transducers

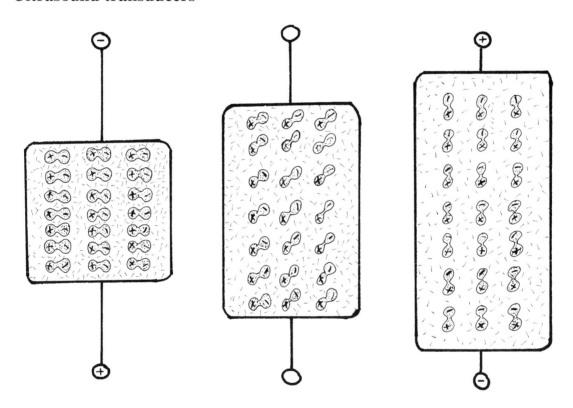

Use the above diagram to answer question 1.049.

1.049 Crystals possessing the piezoelectric effect have molecular dipoles which are:
    A. randomly ordered
    B. aligned
    C. alternating
    D. changing direction constantly

B is correct.
The piezoelectric effect describes the use of substances that have negative and positive poles. For this effect to be enabled, the positives must be positioned in the same geometric direction and the negatives positioned in the opposite direction. This arrangement is also termed 'aligned dipoles'.

1.050 The minimum axial resolution is approximately equal to:
A. spatial pulse length
B. wavelength
C. 1/2 spatial pulse length
D. beam diameter

C is correct.
The axial resolution describes the minimum distance that the ultrasound imager is able to resolve along the axis of the beam. This resolution is dependent upon spatial pulse length. The pulse has to produce echoes for two closely spaced reflectors without the returning echoes being superimposed. This can only occur at a distance ≥ 1/2 spatial pulse length.

1.051 The ability to discriminate between two closely spaced reflectors is known as:
A. definition
B. range accuracy
C. resolution
D. amplification

C is correct.
There are two types of resolution – detail and contrast. Detail resolution is subdivided into three categories: axial, lateral and slice thickness. Detail resolution is the ability to resolve closely spaced objects.

1.052 Of the following, the transducer of choice for deep abdominal scanning would be:
A. small diameter, low frequency,
B. large diameter, high frequency
C. large diameter, low frequency
D. medium diameter, medium frequency
E. small diameter, high frequency

C is correct.
To image deep in the abdomen, a low-frequency transducer crystal should be selected as this provides the best penetration. A large-diameter transducer crystal has a longer near zone than that of a smaller-diameter crystal. The near zone is the part of the ultrasound beam that has the best focus. A larger-diameter crystal also has less divergence or spreading of the beam in the far zone than a small-diameter crystal. These two qualities make a larger-diameter transducer the better choice for deep abdominal scanning.

1.053 The piezoelectric effect will be exhibited only by:
A. metallic materials
B. crystalline properties
C. natural materials
D. ceramic material

B is correct.
Quartz, Rochelle salts and PZT (lead, zirconate, titanate) are materials that exhibit the piezoelectric effect. Some are natural (quartz, Rochelle salts) and some are man-made (PZT), but all piezoelectric materials are crystalline.

1.054 Which of the following can be accomplished by phased array?
A. beam-shaping
B. beam-focusing
C. beam-steering
D. all of the above

D is correct.
The phased-array transducer setup is the most versatile of all transducers. This arrangement of crystals can shape, steer and focus the beam.

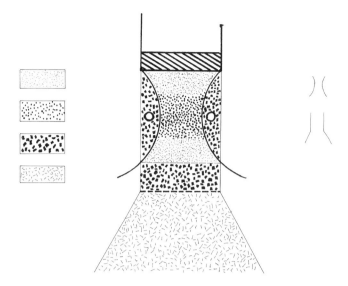

Use the above diagram to answer question 1.055.

1.055 The effect of focusing is:
    A. improved lateral resolution
    B. improved axial resolution
    C. decreased beam width
    D. A and B
    E. A and C

E is correct.
Focusing the ultrasound beam involves narrowing the beam via an external lens or a curved crystal. Making the beam narrower improves the lateral resolution.

1.056 Wavelength is determined by:
    A. crystal thickness
    B. crystal manufacture
    C. the source
    D. the medium
    E. all of the above
    F. C and D only

E is correct.
The beam frequency is influenced by crystal thickness and, thus, its manufacture. If the crystal is thinner, then the beam frequency is higher. The beam frequency and the propagation speed of the medium determine the final beam wavelength. Thus, a 5-MHz beam will have a different wavelength in soft tissue than it has in bone.

1.057 Lateral resolution can be improved by:
    A. reducing the beam diameter
    B. focusing
    C. eliminating side lobes
    D. all of the above

D is correct.
Lateral resolution is determined by beam width. Focusing, reducing the beam diameter, and eliminating side lobes will improve lateral resolution.

1.058 Longitudinal resolution cannot be improved by:
    A. increasing frequency
    B. increasing wavelength
    C. more damping
    D. A and B

B is correct.
Longitudinal resolution is another name for axial resolution. Axial resolution is improved by reducing the spatial pulse length, which can be shortened by damping, or by increasing the frequency, which will decrease the wavelength. With a constant number of cycles, a reduction in wavelength effectively decreases the spatial pulse length.

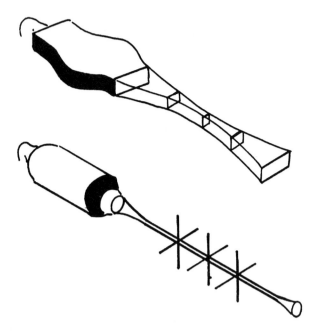

Use the above diagram to answer question 1.059.

1.059 Linear and annular arrays are:
   A. sector scanners
   B. real-time multielement instruments
   C. Doppler-only systems
   D. always equipped with fixed focal zones

B is correct.
This question requires that both types of transducer satisfy the answer; therefore, both are real-time multielement instruments.

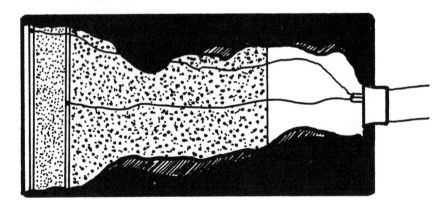

Use the above diagram to answer question 1.060.

1.060 The transducer backing material:
   A. lowers the Q (quality) factor
   B. reduces ring-down artifact
   C. ensures a shorter pulse
   D. all of the above

D is correct.
The transducer backing material is used primarily to reduce excessive ringing. The amount of ringing is known as the Q factor. A lowered Q factor means a shorter pulse.

1.061 Transducers should be steam-sterilized:
A. at least once a year
B. when required
C. never
D. at least monthly

C is correct.
Steam-sterilization is a harsh, yet effective, technique. However, transducers are too delicate to be steam-sterilized.

1.062 Bandwidth signifies:
A. source of artifact
B. potential shade of gray
C. a range of frequencies produced by a single transducer element
D. undesirable interference or noise

C is correct.
The beam bandwidth describes the range of frequencies produced by the ultrasound beam.

1.063 The operating frequency of the transducer is NOT dependent upon:
A. crystal thickness
B. crystal diameter
C. crystal resonance
D. crystal manufacture specifications

B is correct.
The manner in which the crystal is made includes its thickness and its resonance characteristics. The crystal diameter influences the beam width.

1.064 Beam diameter is NOT dependent upon:
A. wavelength
B. frequency
C. transducer diameter
D. distance from the transducer
E. intensity

E is correct.
The beam diameter is dependent upon the length of the near zone, focusing and the frequency of the transducer. The intensity does not influence the diameter.

1.065 Increasing the _____ decreases the beam diameter in the _____:
A. frequency, far zone
B. wavelength, near zone
C. intensity, near zone
D. intensity, far zone

A is correct.
Equations that relate the near zone length, the angle of divergence and the crystal diameter can thus be summarized: If the crystal diameter is increased, with constant frequency, the near field is lengthened and the far zone will not diverge as much. Also, as the beam frequency is increased, with a fixed-diameter crystal, the near zone is lengthened and the far zone will not diverge as much.

1.066 The smaller the distance detected between reflectors:
A. the worse the resolution
B. the better the resolution
C. the larger the reflector
D. the weaker the echo

B is correct.
Resolution refers to the ability to see fine detail. An improvement in visualizing fine detail is an improvement in resolution.

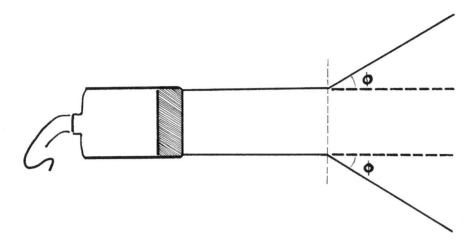

Use the above diagram to answer question 1.067.

1.067 The Fraunhofer zone is marked by:
    A. two focal zones
    B. two near zone lengths
    C. the angle of divergence
    D. less attenuation

C is correct.
The Fraunhofer zone is the same as the far field, and begins at the focal point and point of beam divergence.

1.068 A transducer's operating frequency is determined by the:
    A. crystal diameter
    B. backing material
    C. excitation voltage amplitude
    D. crystal thickness

D is correct.
Most transducers match the voltage frequency to the crystal's nominal or resonant frequency. However, the frequency is determined by crystal thickness.

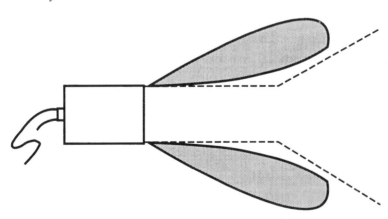

Use the above diagram to answer question 1.069.

1.069 Extraneous energy components that are NOT part of the primary beam are:
    A. acoustic shadows
    B. reverberations
    C. tangent wavefronts
    D. side lobes

D is correct.
Side lobes are energy components alongside the main beam.

1.070 The device that generates ultrasound energy is the:
   A. receiver
   B. pulser
   C. transducer

C is correct.
The term 'transducer' means 'to lead across' and is used to describe a device that transforms one form of energy to another. The crystal or transducer transforms electrical energy into mechanical or sound energy.

1.071 Transducers may be the source of a potential electrical hazard because the applied voltages may be as high as:
   A. 5 V
   B. 500 V
   C. 10,000 V

B is correct.
A cracked or broken cord between the transducer and the ultrasound unit can deliver an electrical shock in the range of 500 V.

1.072 A highly damped transducer has:
   A. poor axial resolution
   B. reduced spatial pulse length
   C. decreased bandwidth
   D. increased Q (quality) factor

B is correct.
The backing material in a transducer setup is used to damp the crystal. Damping the crystal means reducing excessive vibration or ringing. This process reduces the spatial pulse length, improves axial resolution, and increases the bandwidth and Q factor.

1.073 Two methods that can be used to focus a single-element transducer are:
   A. internal or external
   B. internal or an acoustic lens
   C. external or a curved crystal
   D. any of the above

D is correct.
'Internal focusing' is a term used to describe a transducer that is concave in shape to focus the beam. Acoustic lenses and other external methods can also be used.

1.074 The length of the near zone:
   A. increases with an increase in frequency
   B. decreases with an increase in crystal diameter
   C. is determined by pulse repetition rate
   D. increases as the wavelength increases

A is correct.
The length of the near zone increases with increased crystal diameter and increased frequency.

1.075 The use of a large-diameter transducer will cause:
   A. a decrease in the near zone length
   B. an axial resolution improvement
   C. a decrease in the angle of divergence
   D. a decrease in the far field intensity

C is correct.
The length of the near zone increases with increased crystal diameter and increased frequency. This method improves the lateral resolution.

1.076 Both axial and lateral resolution will improve by:
   A. using a smaller-diameter transducer
   B. using a higher-frequency transducer
   C. increasing the power output
   D. all of the above

B is correct.
Although both increased frequency and increased crystal diameter will decrease both beam width and angle of divergence, only an increase in frequency improves both axial and lateral resolution. An increased frequency can decrease the spatial pulse length (improving axial resolution) and an increased frequency can increase the near zone length (improving lateral resolution).

1.077 Normally, axial resolution:
   A. is better than longitudinal resolution
   B. is poorer than the azimuthal resolution
   C. is better than the lateral resolution
   D. is poorer than the depth resolution

C is correct.
In general, the size of the pulse is smaller than the width of the beam; thus, axial resolution is always better than lateral resolution.

1.078 The axial resolution is determined by spatial pulse length.
  A. true
  B. false

A is correct.
The size of the pulse directly influences what the pulse can fit in between and thus affects the system's axial resolution.

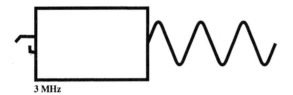

3 MHz

●

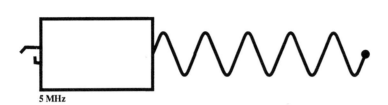

5 MHz

Use the above diagram to answer question 1.079.

1.079 The axial resolution from a 5.0-MHz transducer that produces a pulse with 3 cycles will be _____ the axial resolution with a 3.0-MHz transducer that produces a pulse with 5 cycles.
  A. the same as
  B. better than
  C. poorer than

B is correct.
A 5.0-MHz crystal produces a smaller wavelength than does a 3.0-MHz crystal. If there are fewer cycles with a 5.0-MHz compared with a 3.0-MHz transducer, then the pulse of the 5.0-MHz transducer will be smaller than that of the 3.0-MHz and, thus, the axial resolution will be better.

1.080 The convex-array transducer produces a sector image. The scanning surface of this transducer is larger than that of the electronic phased array. A disadvantage of the electronic phased array is:
  A. higher cost
  B. lack of electronic focusing
  C. duplex operation is not possible

A is correct.
The technology needed to have variable timing in the electronic phased array makes it more expensive together with the fact that the individual crystal must be matched so that they work together. Remember that, with a phased-array system, the collection of crystals works together to produce one pulse whereas, with a convex array, one or two crystals work together to produce one pulse.

1.081 The acoustic impedance of the transducer's matching layer:
  A. is chosen to have increased internal reflections
  B. is chosen to improve transmission into the body
  C. determines the frequency
  D. none of the above

B is correct.
The matching layer of the transducer is designed to match the impedances of the crystal and the soft tissue of the body.

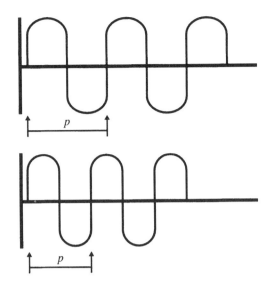

Use the above diagram to answer question 1.082.

1.082 If there is an increase in transducer frequency, the period:
    A. increases
    B. decreases
    C. stays the same

B is correct.
Frequency and period are reciprocal. Therefore, when one is increased, the other is decreased.

1.083 If there is an increase in transducer frequency, the pulse duration:
    A. increases
    B. decreases
    C. stays the same

B is correct.
An increase in frequency causes a decrease in wavelength. This, in turn, decreases both the spatial pulse length and pulse duration.

1.084 If there is an increase in transducer frequency, the spatial pulse length:
    A. increases
    B. decreases
    C. stays the same

B is correct.
The frequency causes an increase in wavelength. This, in turn, decreases both the spatial pulse length and pulse duration.

1.085 If there is an increase in transducer frequency, the PRF:
    A. increases
    B. decreases
    C. stays the same

C is correct.
PRF stands for 'pulse repetition frequency'. This refers to the number of pulses emitted by the transducer per second. This, however, is not related to the transducer frequency.

1.086 If the amount of damping decreases, the period:
    A. increases
    B. decreases
    C. stays the same

C is correct.
Damping refers to a method of shortening the ultrasound pulse length by reducing the number of cycles produced. This, however, is not related to the transducer period.

1.087 If the amount of damping decreases, the Q factor:
   A. increases
   B. decreases
   C. stays the same

A is correct.
Damping is used to reduce excessive ringing. This decreases or degrades the quality. The reverse is also true.

1.088 If the amount of damping decreases, the spatial pulse length:
   A. increases
   B. decreases
   C. stays the same

A is correct.
Damping is used to reduce ringing, thereby shortening the pulse.

1.089 If the amount of damping decreases, the bandwidth:
   A. increases
   B. decreases
   C. stays the same

B is correct.
Damping reduces crystal ringing and, in effect, increases the variety of different frequencies present. If there is a greater variety of frequencies, there is an increase in, or widerning of, the bandwidth.

1.090 If the amount of damping decreases, the number of cycles:
   A. increases
   B. decreases
   C. stays the same

A is correct.
Damping effectively decreases the number of cycles present in any one pulse.

Pulse-echo instruments

1.091 The average power output of diagnostic pulsed ultrasound is usually in the range of:
   A. 1–100 W
   B. 10–20 W
   C. 50–100 W
   D. 1–100 mW

D is correct.
Although some current ultrasound units (in particular, modes such as pulse-wave Doppler) have very high power outputs, the average range is usually up to 100 mW.

1.092 The pulse length increases:
   A. as frequency increases
   B. as the Q factor increases
   C. as axial resolution increases
   D. two of the above

B is correct.
The Q factor describes how much the crystal continues to vibrate after being stimulated. The higher the Q factor, the longer the vibration lasts, the more cycles are present and, therefore, the longer the pulse.

1.093 The weakest echoes are eliminated from the display by use of:
   A. suppression-rejection
   B. time-gain compensation
   C. depth-gain compensation

A is correct.
Time-gain compensation and depth-gain compensation are methods of increasing the amplitude of the received echoes once they are in the receiver.

1.094 Factors that determine echo location on a display include: I, position of the transducer (from static imaging); II, direction towards which the beam is traveling; III, time delay between pulse generation and reception of the echo; IV, assumed velocity of sound in soft tissue.
A. I, II, III
B. I, III
C. II, IV
D. I, II, III, IV

D is correct.
The position of the transducer, beam direction, the time delay and velocity of sound determine the echo location.

1.095 The number of cycles in a pulse may be reduced by:
A. increasing the TGC
B. increasing the damping
C. increasing the frequency
D. none of the above

B is correct.
Damping reduces the number of cycles in a pulse.

1.096. With pulse ultrasound, the transducer is active _____% of the time.
A. 1
B. 15
C. 25
D. 50

A is correct.
With pulse ultrasound, the system spends the majority of its time listening to or receiving the returned echoes. Very little time (< 1%) is spent producing the ultrasound pulse.

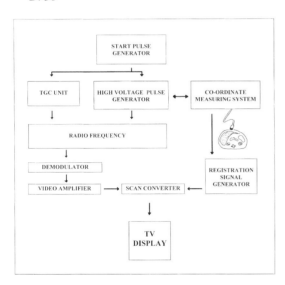

Use the above diagram to answer question 1.097.

1.097 The response of the entire ultrasound system is initiated and synchronized by the:
A. transducer
B. receiver
C. pulser
D. processor
E. none of the above

D is correct.
The master synchronizer or computer processor is responsible for coordinating all functions of the ultrasound unit.

1.098 The ratio of the largest-to-smallest power that an ultrasound system can handle is known as:
   A. time-gain compensation
   B. decibels
   C. dynamic range
   D. compression

C is correct.
The dynamic range is defined as the ratio between the largest and smallest powers that can be handled by the system.

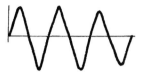 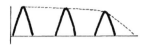 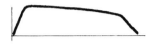

Use the above diagram to answer question 1.099.

1.099 Demodulation is accomplished by:
   A. damping
   B. rectification and smoothing
   C. rejection and suppression
   D. time-gain compensation

B is correct.
Demodulation is a simple way to describe signal processing of the RF signal. Demodulation consists of the removal of negative components and contouring of the signal. This process is also called rectification and smoothing.

1.100 Amplification is an operation performed by the:
   A. pulser
   B. transducer
   C. receiver
   D. scan converter
   E. display

C is correct.
When the return echoes enter the system, they are very weak. They must be boosted in power to be handled by the system. This is called amplification.

1.101 The lower the frequency, the:
   A. longer the spatial pulse length (SPL)
   B. better the longitudinal resolution
   C. deeper the penetration
   D. less the attenuation per centimeter
   E. A, C and D only

E is correct.
The lower the frequency, the longer the SPL, the deeper the penetration and the less the attenuation. A higher frequency would improve the longitudinal resolution.

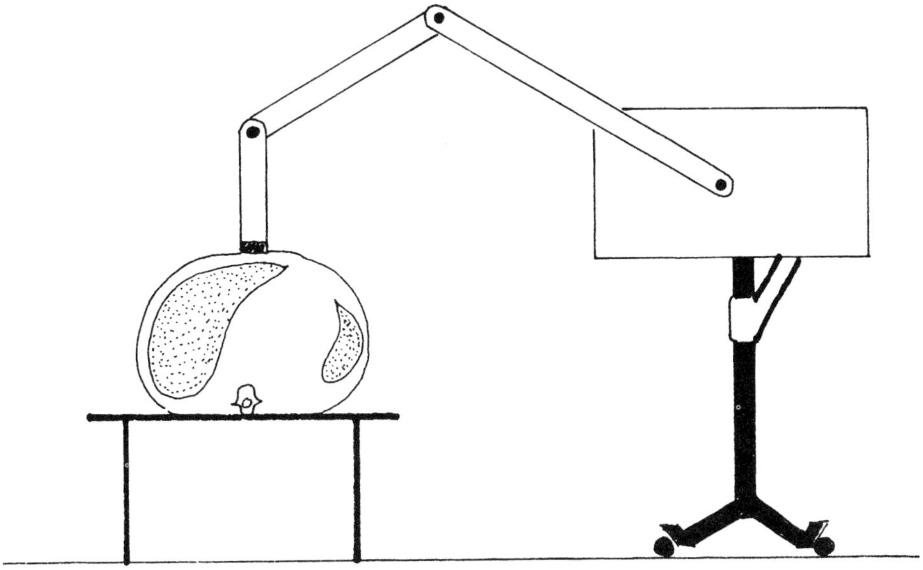

Use the above diagram to answer question 1.102.

1.102 Echo location information is transmitted by an articulated-arm B scanner via:
  A. potentiometers
  B. the receiver
  C. the display
  D. strong reflectors

A is correct.
This question refers to the articulated B scanner where the location of the transducer arm is determined by the angles at each joint of the arm. The sensors that determine the joint angle are called potentiometers.

1.103 The resolution capabilities of the system are mainly functions of the:
  A. pulser
  B. transducer
  C. receiver
  D. display

B is correct.
The resolution of the system is determined by crystal thickness, crystal diameter and pulse length. These characteristics are determined by the transducer.

1.104 The ability of a system to detect weak reflectors is:
  A. amplification
  B. amplitude
  C. TGC
  D. sensitivity

D is correct.
Sensitivity refers to the system's ability to detect and display information. Weak echoes are the most difficult to detect; this is referred to as system sensitivity.

1.105 Increasing the power, in effect, causes an increase in system sensitivity (the ability of a system to detect weaker reflectors).
  A. true
  B. false

A is correct.
Increasing the power in a system increases the strength of the reflection, thus rendering weak echoes considerably stronger so that echoes that would normally be too weak to be displayed can be visualized.

1.106 Increasing the pulser voltage does not increase the power output of the transducer.
   A. true
   B. false

B is correct.
Power equals amplitude squared; therefore, increasing power must increase any unit of amplitude which includes, for example, voltage or density pressure.

1.107 Which of the following is NOT a general ultrasound instrumentation component?
   A. master synchronizer
   B. pulser/transmitter
   C. transducer
   D. interpolator

D is correct.
The primary components of an ultrasound instrument include the master synchronizer, pulser, transmitter and transducer. There is no such ultrasound device as an interpolator.

1.108 Which of the five receiver functions deals with the machine's ability to reduce the total range from the smallest to the largest signal?
   A. compensation
   B. compression
   C. rejection

B is correct.
The question is the definition of compression.

1.109 One component of demodulation is rectification and the other is:
   A. rejection
   B. compensation
   C. smoothing

C is correct.
Demodulation is a simplified way of describing signal processing. The two basic components are rectification and smoothing.

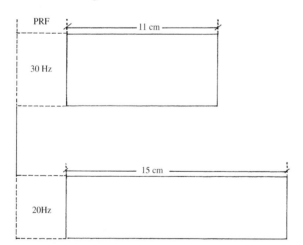

Use the above diagram to answer question 1.110.

1.110 As the imaging depth increases, the PRF:
   A. increases
   B. decreases
   C. remains the same

B is correct.
PRF stands for 'pulse repetition frequency'. The unit will be able to send more pulses per unit of time if the depth of field is shorter; therefore, the PRF decreases with increasing depth.

1.111 The pulse duration will increase if the period:
    A. increases
    B. decreases
    C. remains the same

A is correct.
The period is the time taken for one cycle. The pulse duration is defined as the period × number of cycles in one pulse. Therefore, if the period increases and the number of cycles remains constant, the pulse duration will increase.

1.112 If all other parameters remain constant, the PRF increases:
    A. if the duty factor increases
    B. if the frequency decreases
    C. if the period increases

A is correct.
PRF stands for 'pulse repetition frequency', which refers to the number of pulses emitted per second. If there are more pulses sent per second, then the transducer is on more of the time; thus, the duty factor increases.

1.113 By adjusting the depth, the operator changes the duty factor.
    A. true
    B. false

A is correct.
The depth of field directly affects the PRF and PRP. The PRF and PRP affect the duty factor.

1.114 The spatial pulse length will increase if the frequency:
    A. increases
    B. decreases
    C. remains the same

B is correct.
Increasing the frequency will decrease the wavelength which, in turn, decreases the spatial pulse length.

1.115 The ultrasound beam is more homogeneous if the spatial peak/spatial average intensity is:
    A. 1
    B. 50%
    C. 0

A is correct.
If the spatial peak and spatial average intensities are the same, the beam is more homogeneous.

1.116 The ultrasound beam is off if the duty factor is:
    A. 1
    B. 100%
    C. 0

C is correct.
The duty factor is the percentage of time that the pulse is on. If the pulse is not on, the duty factor is 0.

Principles of pulse-echo imaging

1.117 Real-time imaging is achieved by:
    A. articulated-arm scanners
    B. mechanically driven transducers
    C. electrically fired arrays
    D. B and C only

D is correct.
The advent of real-time has brought about a dramatic improvement in ultrasound imaging. Fetal movement can now be seen when it occurs. This was only possible with non-manual scanning setups using mechanical and electronic transducers.

1.118 A common frame rate for real-time equipment is:
    A. 5/s
    B. 25/s
    C. 50/s
    D. 100/s

B is correct.
The frame rate has to be high to reduce flicker and produce what appears to be a real-time image. The real-time equipment today creates 'odd' and 'even' fields. Each field is created in 1/60th of a second. Most single frames are updated 25–30 times a second.

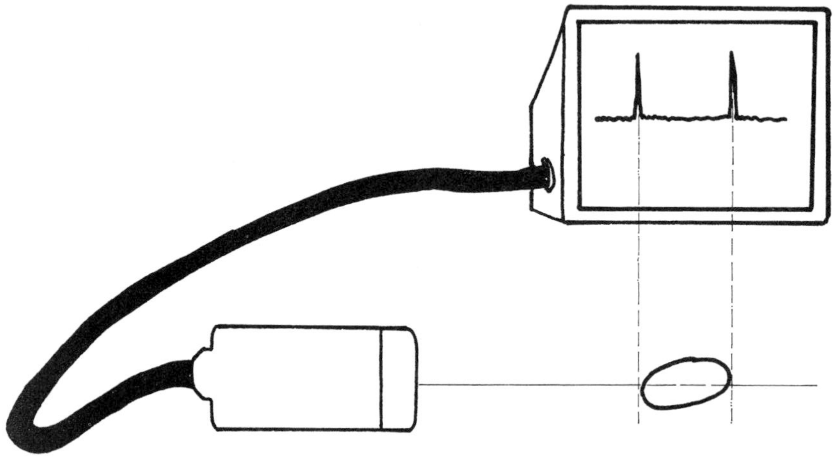

Use the above diagram to answer question 1.119.

1.119 The magnitude of the echo is related to the height of the spike (deflection) in:
  A. A-mode
  B. B-mode
  C. M-mode
  D. all of the above

A is correct.
The amplitude (A-mode) is so named because it is a graphic presentation in which the height of the spike represents the strength of the echo.

1.120 The major benefit of using a water path is:
  A. the speed of sound is increased
  B. reverberation is increased
  C. the dead zone is eliminated from the area of interest
  D. it is cheaper and less complicated than phased array

C is correct.
The water path pulls the transducer away from the skin surface without attenuating the beam. This technique renders superficial structures more easily seen.

1.121 A-mode differs from M-mode in that:
  A. A-mode is unrectified
  B. only A-mode displays reflector motion
  C. M-mode reflects echo amplitude whereas A-mode does not
  D. none of the above are true

D is correct.
A-mode stands for 'amplitude mode' and M-mode stands for 'motion mode'.

1.122 A real-time frame rate of 50 frames/s will produce _____ scan lines if the PRF is 1000 Hz.
  A. 10
  B. 20
  C. 50
  D. 1000

B is correct.
PRF = frame rate × number of scan lines.

1.123 The number of horizontal scan lines in a normal television frame is:
  A. 262
  B. 525
  C. 60
  D. 30

B is correct.
The normal TV frame has a standard 525 horizontal lines.

1.124 The number of TV frames/s is:
    A. 10
    B. 30
    C. 60
    D. 512

B is correct.
The TV frame is made up of horizontal lines that are placed on the screen via a raster pattern. The odd-numbered lines are placed first, then the even-numbered lines. The odd frame is completed in 1/60th of a second followed by making of the even field. This process reduces image flicker. Thus, making both the odd- and even-numbered fields to complete a frame takes 1/30th of a second.

1.125 An electronic phased array always produces a sector image.
    A. true
    B. false

A is correct.
All phased-array transducers produce sector-image formats.

1.126 Annular-array transducers use mechanical beam-steering.
    A. true
    B. false

A is correct.
The annular-array transducer involves crystals arranged in concentric rings. This pattern can produce remarkable focus, but its geometry prevents scanning. Therefore, the beam has to be mechanically scanned.

1.127 Annular-array transducers cannot be electronically focused.
    A. true
    B. false

B is correct.
The annular-array transducer involves an arrangement of crystals in concentric rings. This produces remarkable focusing by stimulating the outer ring first and then the innermost rings.

1.128 Frequency shift is normally detected with a static B scanner.
    A. true
    B. false

B is correct.
The static B scanner cannot produce frequency-shift information.

1.129 Which of the following display modes has time as one of its axes?
    A. A-mode
    B. B-mode
    C. C-mode
    D. M-mode

D is correct.
Only the motion (M)-mode and the Doppler mode use time as an axis.

1.130 Dynamic focusing can only be accomplished with mechanical scanning.
    A. true
    B. false

B is correct.
Dynamic focusing is one of the advantages of a phased-array format. The phased-array format allows intricate manipulation of crystal excitation.

1.131 If the PRF is 1 kHz, what will the maximum imaging depth be?
    A. 20 cm
    B. 50 cm
    C. 1540 cm
    D. 77 cm

D is correct.
The relationship between imaging depth and PRF is maximum depth = 77 cm/PRF (kHz).

Given: 5 = number of focuses

20 = frame rate

2000 = PRF

Required: Lines per frame

Solution: (number of focuses) (frame rate) (lines per frame) = PRF

(5) (20) (lines per frame) = 2000

$$\frac{100 \text{ (lines per frame)} = 2000}{100}$$

lines per frame = 20

Use the above diagram to answer question 1.132.

1.132 If the number of focuses is 5 and the frame rate is 20 frames/s, approximately what is the maximum permitted number of lines/frame to avoid ambiguity with a PRF of 2000?

    A. 20

    B. 200

    C. 40

    D. 400

A is correct.
The PRF is equal to the number of focuses × lines/frame × frame rate.

1.133 Using established equations, if the PRF is 1 kHz, the frame rate is 25/s and the rectangular display width is 10 cm, what is the line density?

    A. 4 lines/cm

    B. 25 lines/cm

    C. 250 lines/cm

A is correct.
The PRF ÷ frame rate = maximum lines/frame.

1.134 The articulated-arm scanner is associated with which pulse-echo technique?

    A. A-mode

    B. B-mode

    C. C-mode

    D. M-mode

B is correct.
The articulated-arm scanner is also called the articulated-arm B scanner. The B scanner is also known as the B-mode scanner.

1.135 B-mode demonstrates brightness on the:

    A. X axis

    B. Y axis

    C. Z axis

C is correct.
A still B-mode image demonstrates depth on the Y axis, length on the X axis, and brightness or amplitude on the Z axis.

1.136 The maximum image depth is _____ to PRF:

    A. directly proportional

    B. inversely proportional

B is correct.
If the maximum image depth is increased, more time is needed for each pulse to travel; therefore, the PRF will be decreased.

1.137 Line density is _____ to the field of view.

    A. directly proportional

    B. inversely proportional

B is correct.
If the field of view is increased, assuming that there is a finite number of lines that can be displayed, the line density will be decreased.

1.138 The C in C-scan stands for:
A. continuous
B. constant
C. compressional

B is correct.
The C stands for 'constant' and refers to the constant depth of this particular imaging technique.

Image storage and display

1.139 A digital scan converter is a:
A. receiver
B. display
C. computer memory
D. cathode ray tube

C is correct.
All scan converters are memory devices that allow for special techniques such as freeze frame. The digital scan converter is a computerized memory system.

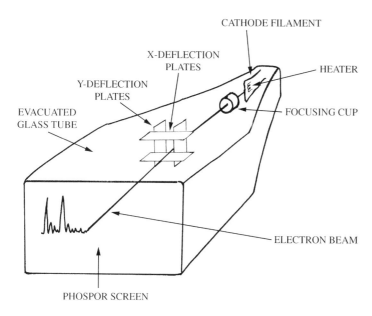

Use the above diagram to answer question 1.140.

1.140 Deflection plates are found in the:
A. receiver
B. pulser
C. preprocessor
D. cathode ray tube

D is correct.
The cathode ray tube was used as a storage device, such as in analog scan converters, and is still used as a display device. The deflection plate directs the electron beam to the screen to draw on it a picture of what is being viewed.

1.141 A television image is constructed by a method known as:
A. Huygen's principle
B. raster scanning
C. scan converting
D. modulation

B is correct.
The raster scanning technique describes the use of a sequence of odd- and even-field display-filling that helps to produce a flicker-free picture.

1.142 The middle-level echo intensity on a gray scale of 32 shades is represented by the binary number:
  A. 10101
  B. 1010
  C. 10000
  D. 11000

C is correct.
The binary system describes how computer memory works. A collection of 0s and 1s is used to indicate on and off commands, respectively. Unlike the decimal system, where each place is counted up to 9 and represents 10 possibilities, each place in the binary system has only two possibilities. From the left, the places are for 1s, followed by 2s, 4s, 8s and so on. This system allows counting up to 16, represented by the binary number 10000.

1.143 The primary purpose of the scan converter is to:
  A. change an analog signal to a digital signal
  B. store an ultrasound image
  C. amplify, compensate and compress
  D. all of the above

B is correct.
All scan converters store information so that it can be converted to a particular display format.

1.144 In relation to small reflectors, pixel size should ideally be:
  A. smaller
  B. larger
  C. the same
  D. inconsequential

A is correct.
The smaller the pixel size, the greater the resolution of the image information will be.

1.145 The information that is normally fed to a scan converter:
  A. contains echo position information
  B. contains echo amplitude information
  C. is analog
  D. all of the above

D is correct.
The scan converter holds all the echo return information. It must therefore be able to determine echo location and strength in the original or analog form before storage.

1.146 Preprocessing of the information that is fed to the scan converter:
  A. enlarges each pixel to provide a magnified image
  B. determines the CRT brightness assigned to stored gray-scale levels
  C. determines the assignment of echoes to predetermined gray levels
  D. determines the gray-scale emphasis of stored gray levels

C is correct.
Preprocessing describes how the information is manipulated before it reaches the scan converter.

1.147 A 7-bit digital memory stores a maximum of 64 shades of gray.
  A. true
  B. false

B is correct.
A 7-bit memory will store the equivalent of 2^7 power, or 128 shades of gray.

1.148 A typical image matrix memory size is 512×512:
  A. true
  B. false

A is correct.
The digital scan convertor uses a matrix of memory location. The number of pixels geometrically is 512×512

1.149 Most real-time ultrasound scanners use analog scan converters.
  A. true
  B. false

B is correct.
With the advent of computers, the digital scan converter flexibility and reliability render the analog scan converter virtually obsolete.

1.150 What type of storage medium is used by videotape recorders?
  A. magnetic
  B. optical
  C. thermal
  D. capacitive

A is correct.
Modern videotape recorders store information on ferrous oxide magnetic strips.

1.150 What type of storage medium is used by videotape recorders?
   A. magnetic
   B. optical
   C. thermal
   D. capacitive

A is correct.
Modern videotape recorders store information on ferrous oxide magnetic strips.

1.151 In a digital scan converter, the _____ receives information from the A to D converter.
   A. digital memory
   B. D to A converter
   C. TV monitor

A is correct.
For a digital memory to be used, the analog signal must be converted into a digital signal, then stored in the digital memory. Afterwards, the digital information is converted back into analog form to be displayed.

1.152 Preprocessing involves manipulating the data before it is stored.
   A. true
   B. false

A is correct.
The definition of preprocessing is to manipulate information before storage by the scan converter.

1.153 The analog scan converter uses an element matrix of:
   A. 1000 × 1000
   B. 512 × 512
   C. 525 × 525

A is correct.
The analog scan converter uses a dielectric matrix with a format of 1000 × 1000.

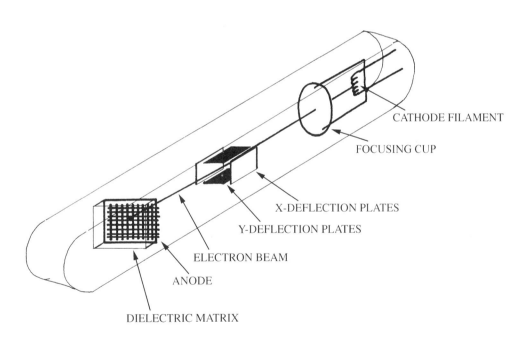

CATHODE FILAMENT

FOCUSING CUP

X-DEFLECTION PLATES

Y-DEFLECTION PLATES

ELECTRON BEAM

ANODE

DIELECTRIC MATRIX

Use the above diagram to answer question 1.154.

1.154 The electronic storage tube is the same as the:
   A. digital scan converter
   B. analog scan converter
   C. preprocessing
   D. postprocessing

B is correct.
The dielectric matrix is also called an electronic storage tube.

Doppler

1.155 A change in frequency caused by reflector motion is known as:
- A. Huygen's principle
- B. Snell's law
- C. the Doppler effect
- D. Schlieren system

C is correct.
The apparent change in frequency is the definition of the Doppler effect.

1.156 The technique used to create the color-flow display is:
- A. FFT
- B. autocorrelation
- C. zero-crossing method

B is correct.
The mathematical technique used to analyze the data is autocorrelation.

1.157 The X axis of the spectral display is divided into:
- A. sampling intervals
- B. sample volumes
- C. gates

A is correct.
The sampling intervals on the spectral display represent the moments in time that frequency information was acquired.

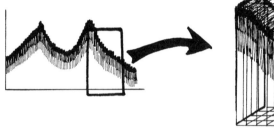 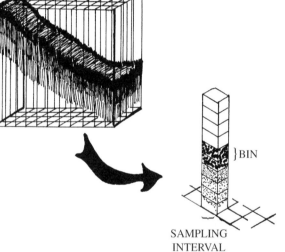

}BIN

SAMPLING
INTERVAL

Use the above diagram to answer question 1.158.

1.158 With Doppler, frequency points are staked into vertical columns called:
- A. pixels
- B. words
- C. bins
- D. bits

C is correct.
The higher the column, the higher the frequency shift. This component is called a bin.

1.159 With Doppler, signal transfer between channels is called:
- A. crosshair
- B. crossbow
- C. crosstalk
- D. crosstown

C is correct.
In systems where there are two channels, information that is ambiguous between the two is called crosstalk.

1.160 The Nyquist limit is equal to:
    A. 1/2 PRF
    B. PRF
    C. 1/2 PRP
    D. PRP

A is correct.
The Nyquist limit is the highest frequency that can be measured under a particular pulsing cycle.

Image features and artifacts

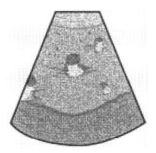

Use the above diagram to answer question 1.161.

1.161 An increase in amplitude from structures that lie behind a weak attenuator is:
    A. reflection
    B. enhancement
    C. artifact
    D. all of the above

B is correct.
Acoustic enhancement describes a strong amplitude behind a weak attenuator.

1.162 Enhancement is caused by:
    A. strong reflectors
    B. improved longitudinal resolution
    C. focusing
    D. increased propagation speed
    E. weak attenuators

E is correct.
Acoustic enhancement describes a strong amplitude behind a weak attenuator.

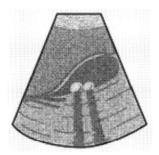

Use the above diagram to answer question 1.163.

1.163 Shadowing:
    A. can be caused by strong reflectors
    B. can cause missing display information
    C. is the result of attenuation
    D. is an absence of transmission
    E. all of the above

E is correct.
Acoustic shadowing is caused by a strong attenuator.

1.164 Artifacts from energy directed far from the main beam axis are known as:
   A. side lobe artifact
   B. reflection artifact
   C. impedance artifact
   D. refraction

A is correct.
Side lobes are spurious energy beams that extend out from the sides of the main beam.

1.165 False echoes are longitudinally misplaced by:
   A. diffraction
   B. refraction
   C. reverberation
   D. reflection

C is correct.
Reverberation is caused by multiple tripping of the pulses. These multiple trips produce false echoes.

1.166 The dead-zone artifact is seen in the posterior portion of the image.
   A. true
   B. false

B is correct.
The dead-zone artifact is created by the main impact of the pulse striking the skin surface.

1.167 The ring-down artifact is thought to be caused by resonance.
   A. true
   B. false

A is correct.
The ring-down artifact is associated with gas bubbles. These bubbles vibrate and become sources of sound production. This vibration is called resonance.

1.168 The comet-tail artifact resembles reverberation.
   A. true
   B. false

A is correct.
The comet-tail artifact is created by reverberation within high-velocity objects such as BB-gun pellets and surgical clips. This multiple reflection produces reverberation-like artifact.

1.169 From a single crystal, the beam profile not being entirely uniform produces the artifact called a(n) _____.
   A. ear lobe
   B. grating lobe
   C. side lobe

C is correct.
The beams extending from the main beam are called grating lobes in multielement probes and side lobes in single-element probes.

1.170 Excess gain in the distal portion of an image is called:
   A. shadowing
   B. reverberation
   C. enhancement

C is correct.
Acoustic enhancement is known as excess brightness behind a weak attenuator.

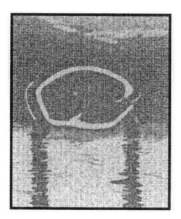

Use the above diagram to answer question 1.171.

1.171 A dropout of echoes posterior to the edge of the fetal skull is largely due to:
  A. refraction
  B. diffraction
  C. ring-down artifact

A is correct.
The curvature of the fetal skull causes the beam to refract and defocus.

1.172 Which of the following artifacts is NOT related to difficulties associated with attenuation?
  A. beam-width
  B. enhancement
  C. mirror-image

A is correct.
A beam-width artifact is a lateral-resolution artifact. This has nothing to do with attenuation.

1.173 'Acoustic speckle' is a resolution artifact:
  A. true
  B. false

A is correct.
The parenchyma of the liver is an artifact. That artifact is called 'acoustic speckle' and is caused by the dispersion pattern of the ultrasound pulses in a particular medium.

1.174 A method of identifying a mirror-image artifact is to change the scanning angle.
  A. true
  B. false

A is correct.
A mirror-image artifact is usually created when there is a strong reflector present. By changing the transducer angle, the mirror-image will move or disappear altogether.

Quality assurance of ultrasound instruments

1.175 System sensitivity can be improved by:
  A. damping
  B. reducing power
  C. increasing gain
  D. eliminating artifact

C is correct.
The ability of the system to detect weak echoes defines system sensitivity. This sensitivity can be improved by increasing system power.

1.176 Registration is the ability to properly reproduce a structure from any angle.
    A. true
    B. false

A is correct.
Placing echoes in the correct location defines registration. This parameter can be tested by ensuring that objects remain in the proper location no matter what angle they are viewed from.

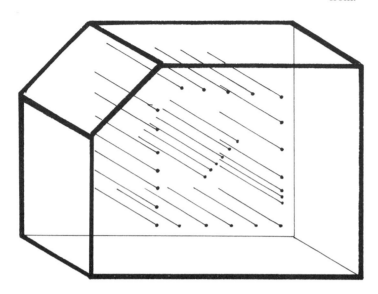

Use the above diagram to answer question 1.177.

1.177 The American Institute of Ultrasound in Medicine (AIUM) 100-mm test object is scanned from:
    A. one plane
    B. two planes
    C. multiple planes

C is correct.
The AIUM 100-mm test object has metal pins arranged in different areas of the object. The pins are assessed at different locations on the test object itself.

1.178 The AIUM 100-mm test object can be used to evaluate the gray scale.
    A. true
    B. false

B is correct.
The AIUM 100-mm test object assesses different geometric parameters of the ultrasound system. By definition, only phantoms are used to assess tissue characteristics.

1.179 The tissue-equivalent test object attenuates ultrasound at approximately 0.004 dB/cm/MHz.
    A. true
    B. false

B is correct.
The tissue-equivalent test object or phantom should have the same attenuation coefficient as soft tissue.

1.180 The AIUM 100-mm test object contains a mixture of ethyl alcohol and:
    A. gel solution
    B. graphite particles
    C. distilled water
    D. mercury

C is correct.
Ethyl alcohol and distilled water, when combined, produces a substance that has a sound velocity similar to that of soft tissue.

Bioeffects and safety

1.181. No significant biological effects have occurred at intensities:
  A. < 100 W/cm^2
  B. < 50 W/ cm^2
  C. < 100 mW/cm^2
  D. < 50 kW/cm^2

C is correct.

The bioeffect standard is still 100 mW/cm^2.

1.182 Biological damage can conceivably be caused by:
  A. heating
  B. cavitation
  C. fluid-streaming
  D. all of the above
  E. A and B only

D is correct.
Heating, cavitation, and fluid-streaming are all categories of bioeffect production.

1.183 The total loss of energy due to reflective and absorptive components is:
  A. heating
  B. friction
  C. reflection
  D. attenuation

D is correct.
Attenuation includes reflection, absorption and scattering. If the frequency is increased, the period is decreased. The period is the pulse duration of one cycle.

1.184 Therefore, it follows that the theoretical possibility of harmful biological effects is NOT increased when power is increased.
  A. true
  B. false

B is correct.
The power output of the ultrasound unit must be assessed as this can increase the possibility of harmful effects.

1.185 Bioeffects from diagnostic ultrasound have NOT been confirmed for intensities below:
  A. 10 mW/cm^2 SPTA
  B. 100 mW/cm^2 SPTA
  C. 1000 mW/cm^2 SPTA
  D. 10,000 mW/cm^2 SPTA

B is correct.
100 mW/cm^2 SPTA is still the AIUM standard.

1.186 Cavitation refers to:
  A. the formation of bubbles
  B. thermal effects of ultrasound
  C. none of the above

A is correct.
Cavitation is the formation of gas bubbles in a liquid medium. The behavior of these bubbles under the influence of a sound field may have destructive effects.

1.187 From a safety standpoint, which one of the following methods is best?
  A. low transmitter output and high receiver gain
  B. high transmitter output and low receiver gain
  C. high near gain and low far gain
  D. low near gain and high far gain
  E. high reject and high transmitter output

A is correct.
The gain of the ultrasound unit is internal. This means that no extra power, intensity or voltage is necessary to increase it. If the power output is increased, more ultrasound energy will enter the medium.

1.188 Is there any knowledge of any bioeffects that ultrasound produces in small animals under experimental conditions?

A. yes

B. no

A is correct.

Many studies have been performed in which there has been some destruction to live animal tissue using ultrasound at differing intensities. These studies cannot be extrapolated to humans and many have not been reproducible.

1.189 Exposure is minimized by using diagnostic ultrasound:

A. only when indicated

B. with minimum intensity

C. with minimum time

D. all of the above

E. none of the above

D is correct.

Exposure will be minimized if less intensity, time and opportunity are implemented.

1.190 Heating depends most directly on:

A. SATA intensity

B. SATP intensity

C. SPTP intensity

A is correct.

Heating is a gradual process that depends on spatial average intensity and temporal average intensity

1.191 There have been no independently confirmed significant biological effects in mammalian tissues exposed *in vivo* to focused ultrasound with intensities below:

A. 100 mW/cm^2

B. 1 W/cm^2

C. 10 mW/cm^2

D. 1 mW/cm^2

B is correct.

The 100 mW/cm^2 rule is applied to unfocused ultrasound whereas 1 W/cm^2 applies to focused ultrasound.

1.192 In which type of cavitation is there bubble formation?

A. transient

B. collapse

C. both

D. mechanical

C is correct.

Both types of cavitation – transient and collapse – involve bubble formation.

1.193 Which form of cavitation is associated with high intensities?

A. stable

B. transient

A is correct.

With stable cavitation, bubble resonance only occurs when the intensity is high.

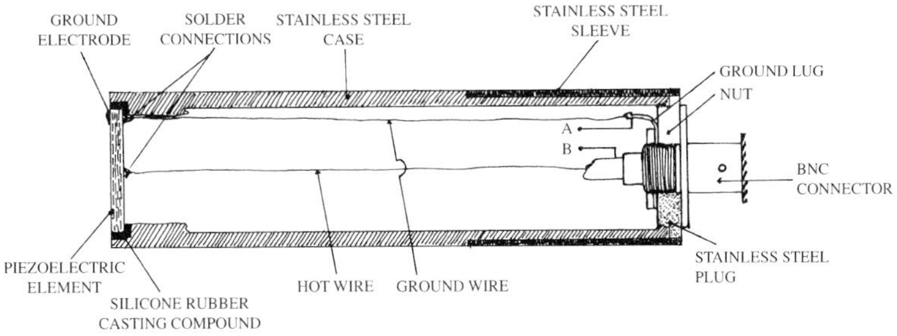

GROUND ELECTRODE   SOLDER CONNECTIONS   STAINLESS STEEL CASE   STAINLESS STEEL SLEEVE   GROUND LUG   NUT   A   B   BNC CONNECTOR   PIEZOELECTRIC ELEMENT   SILICONE RUBBER CASTING COMPOUND   HOT WIRE   GROUND WIRE   STAINLESS STEEL PLUG

Use the above diagram to answer question 1.194.

1.194 Because of its small size, a hydrophone can measure spatial details of a sound beam.
   A. true
   B. false

A is correct.
The hydrophone looks like a small transducer and is sensitive enough to detect the location as well as the strength of the sound pressure.

1.195 Average intensity can be measured by:
   A. hydrophone
   B. force balance
   C. oscilloscope
   D. AIUM test object

A is correct.
The hydrophone measures the average, not the maximum, intensity.

1.196 Some studies of ultrasound bioeffects are performed *in vivo*. What does this term mean?
   A. observable in a living body
   B. observations based on an experiment
   C. discernible in a test tube
   D. perceptible in a plant

A is correct.
Some ultrasound studies are performed on non-living matter and some are performed on live animals.

1.197 The available epidemiological data are sufficient to make a final judgement on the safety of diagnostic ultrasound.
   A. true
   B. false

B is correct.
There are too many parameters and not enough studies to provide conclusive information on ultrasound bioeffects.

1.198 The AIUM considers an ultrasound-induced biological tissue-temperature rise of $< 1°$ C above normal body temperature as safe for clinical studies.
   A. true
   B. false

A is correct.
Temperature rises $\geq 1.5°$ C are likely to have deleterious effects on the human body.

1.199 Of the following choices, which variable is considered the most important for the sonographer with regard to bioeffects?
   A. PRF
   B. frequency
   C. duration of study

C is correct.
The power output of the ultrasound unit is varied by the operator but, on most systems, the actual intensity is not known. The duration or length of study, however, is known.

1.200 Results from experiments *in vitro* serve as a basis for the design of experiments *in vivo*.
   A. true
   B. false

A is correct.
Yes, experiments *in vitro* are used to design experiments *in vivo*.

SECTION 2: THE ABDOMEN (AND SMALL PARTS)

Normal liver

2.001 A sonogram of a normal liver should display:
   A. heterogeneous echogenicity
   B. smooth contour and regions of bull's-eye foci
   C. homogeneous echogenicity interspersed with fluid-filled vessels
   D. homogeneous echogenicity throughout

C is correct.
In a healthy liver, the parenchyma, composed mostly of hepatocytes, displays a moderately echogenic pattern from the anterior portion to the diaphragm. The hepatic veins, portal veins, and large biliary ducts are filled with fluid and are anechoic.

2.002 The portal veins are distinguishable from the hepatic veins in the liver because the:
   A. hepatic veins increase in caliber towards the diaphragm
   B. portal veins display hypoechoic walls and hepatic veins display echogenic walls
   C. portal veins empty into the inferior vena cava (IVC)
   D. portal veins course intrasegmentally whereas the hepatic veins course intersegmentally
   E. A and D
   F. A and C
   G. B and C

E is correct.
The main portal vein is located in the porta hepatis, anterior to the inferior vena cava (IVC). It divides into right and left portal veins, which branch throughout the liver. The walls of the portal veins appear echogenic as they are encased in a collagenous sheath.

2.003 Which of the following is TRUE concerning the caliber of these vessels?
   A. The caliber of the hepatic veins increases as they course towards the diaphragm and IVC
   B. the caliber of the hepatic veins decreases as they course towards the diaphragm and IVC
   C. the caliber of the portal veins is largest at the porta hepatis
   D. the caliber of the portal veins is smallest at the porta hepatis.
   E. A, B and C
   F. A and C
   G. C and D

F is correct.
The portal and hepatic vessels have different branching patterns: the portal veins are largest at the porta hepatis and then divide like the branches of a tree whereas the hepatic veins are like the tributaries of a river that get larger and larger until they join the IVC.

2.004 In the new classification of lobes of the liver:
   A. there are only two lobes, the right and the left
   B. the division between the right and left lobes is through the main lobar fissure
   C. the division between the right and left lobes is where the ligamentum teres is found
   D. the division between the right and left lobes is where the ligamentum venosum is located

B is correct.
In the new classification, there are three lobes: right, left, and caudate. The 'quadrate' lobe is now classified as the medial segment of the left lobe. The division between right and left lobes is through the main lobar fissure, which is localized by the middle hepatic vein superiorly and the gallbladder fossa more inferiorly.

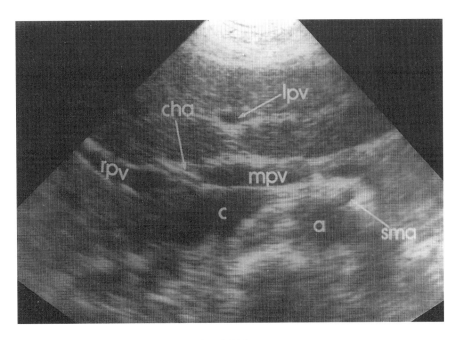

Use the above scan to answer question 2.005.

2.005 The porta hepatis region of the liver seen in this scan represents a:
    A. transverse midline view
    B. right oblique view
    C. midline sagittal view
    D. right parasagittal view

A is correct.

2.006 The ligamentum teres is:
    A. a remnant of the ductus venosus and courses in the main lobar fissure
    B. a remnant of the umbilical vein and courses in the left intersegmental fissure
    C. a remnant of the ductus arteriosus and courses in the left intersegmental fissure
    D. a remnant of the umbilical vein and courses in the main lobar fissure

B is correct.
The ligamentum teres may recanalize into a vein in cases of portal hypertension, thus allowing collateral blood flow from the portal system to the systemic veins of the anterior abdominal wall.

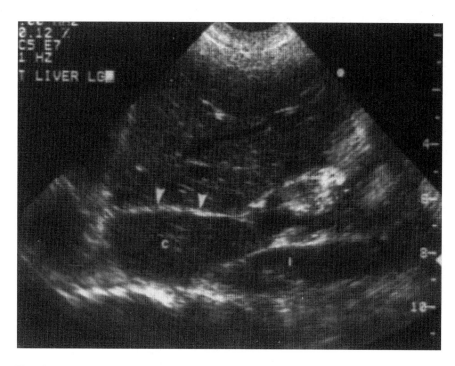

Use the above scan to answer question 2.007.

2.007 In this sonogram of the right upper quadrant, the ligamentum venosum is seen dividing the:
    A. right and left lobes of the liver
    B. caudate and medial segments of the left lobe
    C. caudate and lateral segments of the left lobe
    D. anterior and posterior segments

C is correct.
The ligamentum venosum is a remnant of the ductus venosus, a vessel that permits oxygenated blood to bypass the liver and flow directly to the IVC.

2.008 The portal triad vessels:
    A. empty directly into a central vein within the liver lobule
    B. all carry oxygenated blood
    C. run interlobularly in the portal canals
    D. can only be found in the porta hepatis

C is correct.
The portal triad vessels visualized at the porta hepatis are the hepatic artery, portal vein and common bile duct. On the microscopic level as arterioles, venules and ductules, they course together in the portal canals between the liver lobules.

2.009 The fossa for the IVC is located:
    A. in the main lobar fissure
    B. in the right intersegmental fissure
    C. in the left intersegmental fissure
    D. within the posterior segment of the right lobe

A is correct.
The IVC fossa is located in the main lobar fissure together with the fossa for the gallbladder.

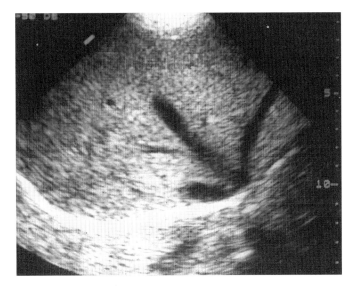

Use the above scan to answer question 2.010.

2.010 The sonographic 'Playboy Bunny' sign seen in this scan is formed by:
    A. right and left branches of the portal vein
    B. right, middle and left hepatic veins draining into the IVC
    C. the cystic duct entering the hepatic duct
    D. the superior mesenteric artery (SMA) branching off from the abdominal aorta

B is correct.
This sign may be imaged subcostally in a superior transverse plane.

2.011 The falciform ligament splits into two layers:
    A. in the porta hepatis region
    B. in the inferoposterior aspect of the liver
    C. on the superior surface of the liver
    D. to form the ligamentum venosum and the ligamentum teres

B is correct.
This can be visualized sonographically only when the liver is surrounded by ascites.

2.012 A scan of the liver labeled L+4 probably demonstrates:
    A. Riedel's lobe
    B. the right lobe and right kidney
    C. the lateral segment of the left lobe
    D. the right portal vein, hepatic artery and biliary duct

D is correct.
L+4 indicates a sagittal scan taken approximately 4 cm to the right of the midline. The structures in the porta hepatis region can be seen.

2.013 Of the following, the BEST way to examine the liver sonographically is to:
    A. turn the patient to the left lateral decubitus (LLD) position and scan during suspended respiration
    B. turn the patient to the right lateral decubitus (RLD) position and scan during suspended respiration
    C. scan the left lobe of the liver intercostally
    D. scan the liver using ONLY a subcostal approach

A is correct.
Scanning with the patient in LLD permits the bowel loops to fall in the opposite direction, thus improving resolution. Suspension of respiration is usually helpful to prevent motion artifact.

2.014 A Riedel's lobe in the liver:
   A. must be evaluated to distinguish it from a mass in the right lobe
   B. connects the caudate and right lobes of the liver
   C. occupies the epigastric region of the abdomen
   D. is a bulbous or tongue-like extension of the right lobe
   E. A and D
   F. B and C

E is correct.
Riedel's lobe, a variant of normal anatomy, is an inferior extension of the anterior and/or posterior segments of the right lobe. It is found more commonly in women.

2.015 The pancreas is more easily visualized when:
   A. the right lobe of the liver is enlarged
   B. when the lateral segment of the left lobe is enlarged
   C. when the caudate lobe is enlarged
   D. when the medial segment of the left lobe is enlarged

B is correct.
An enlarged lateral segment of the left lobe, with sinusoids filled with blood, provides an acoustic window through which to view the pancreas which lies posterior in the abdomen.

2.016 The optimal technique to employ when imaging the liver is to:
   A. always use a low-frequency transducer with a far focus to reach the right hemidiaphragm
   B. always use a high-frequency transducer to get the best resolution of the hepatic parenchyma
   C. use a transducer with the highest frequency possible that penetrates adequately
   D. use a transducer with a short focus to best image the right lobe

C is correct.
In an ultrasound examination, a sonographer must strike a balance between higher-frequency transducers, which give the best resolution, and lower-frequency transducers, which are capable of greater penetration. The focus used in examination of the liver is usually medium, but this depends on the objective of the examination. Some equipment have dynamic focusing, in which all regions of the scan are in focus.

2.017 To scan the liver:
   A. the patient must be NPO for 6–8 hours
   B. the patient must ingest contrast material
   C. the sonographer must scan using only the subcostal technique
   D. the sonographer must scan using only the intercostal technique
   E. no patient preparation is necessary if the examination is focused specifically at the liver

E is correct.
Both subcostal and/or intercostal scanning may be used to visualize the liver, the position of which may vary. If the gallbladder and extrahepatic biliary system are also to be investigated, the patient should then be NPO for 6–8 hours prior to scanning.

2.018 A liver scan is usually performed:
   A. in deep inspiration to move the liver more superiorly
   B. in deep inspiration to bring as much of the liver as possible below the costal margin
   C. using the Valsalva maneuver
   D. with the patient positioned in RLD

B is correct.

2.019 Hepatomegaly is suspected when:
   A. the liver measures > 8 cm in anterior–posterior view
   B. when the liver measures > 14 cm in length
   C. when the right lobe of the liver measures 15–17 cm in length
   D. when the right lobe is palpated below the costal margin
   E. A, B and C
   F. A and B
   G. C and D

G is correct.
Liver size may be assessed by measuring the length of the right lobe, but is best estimated by looking at both sagittal and transverse images.

2.020 In color Doppler scanning of the liver, using the red/towards and blue/away scheme:
   A. portal venous flow will always be displayed in red and hepatic veins in blue
   B. portal venous flow will always be displayed in blue and hepatic veins in red
   C. because color assignment depends on flow direction in relation to the transducer, the portal and hepatic veins may be either red or blue
   D. the common bile duct will be displayed in red
   E. the common bile duct will be displayed in blue

C is correct.
For example, the main portal vein is usually displayed in red whereas the right portal vein may be displayed in blue. Biliary ducts are not blood vessels and do not display color.

Gallbladder and biliary ducts

2.021 NPO for 6–8 hours is recommended for gallbladder scanning because:
   A. the gallbladder cannot be visualized if the patient eats
   B. the right lobe of the liver is better visualized in this state
   C. fasting allows for maximum distention of the gallbladder and extrahepatic biliary ducts
   D. fasting gets rid of bowel gas in the epigastrium

C is correct.
Patients 'fasting' for days or on total parenteral nutrition (TPN) usually display distended gallbladders.

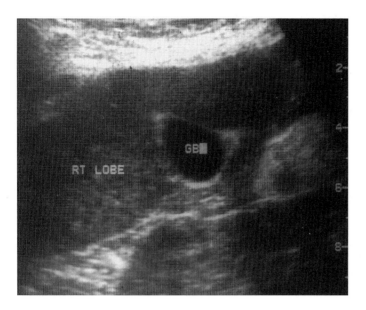

Use the scan above to answer question 2.022.

2.022 In this sonogram, the:
    A. gallbladder is seen in long axis
    B. gallbladder is seen in short axis
    C. gallbladder and cystic duct are both visualized
    D. gallbladder and common bile duct are visualized

B is correct.
In short-axis view, the gallbladder has a rounded contour.

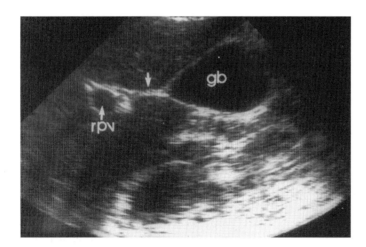

Use the above scan to answer question 2.023.

2.023 In this sonogram, a helpful anatomic landmark to help locate a small contracted gallbladder is the:
    A. ligamentum teres
    B. ligamentum venosum
    C. falciform ligament
    D. main lobar fissure

D is correct.
The gallbladder lies in the fossa delineated by the main lobar fissure.

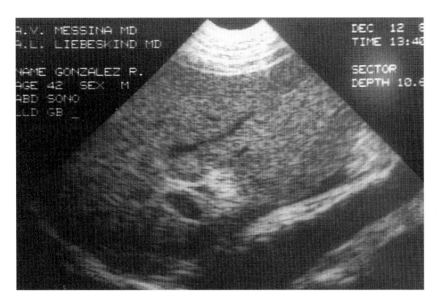

Use the above scan to answer question 2.024.

2.024 At the porta hepatis, this sonogram demonstrates the :
   A. hepatic artery in short axis, right portal vein in long axis, and common hepatic duct in long axis
   B. hepatic artery in short axis, right portal vein in long axis, and common bile duct in short axis
   C. hepatic artery in long axis, main portal vein in short axis and common bile duct in long axis
   D. hepatic artery in short axis, main portal vein in long axis, and common hepatic duct in long axis

A is correct.
Within the substance of the liver, the common hepatic duct can be visualized in the long axis. Extrahepatically, after uniting with the cystic duct, it forms the common bile duct.

2.025 The 'hepatic artery' seen in the above sonogram is the:
   A. common hepatic artery
   B. right hepatic artery
   C. proper hepatic artery
   D. left hepatic artery

B is correct.
The common hepatic artery arises from the celiac axis. After giving rise to the gastroduodenal artery, it is termed the 'proper' hepatic artery. This usually gives rise to the right gastric artery, then bifurcates into the right and left hepatic arteries near the porta hepatis.

2.026 Gallbladder examinations should be done:
   A. with the patient in the supine position only
   B. with the patient in the left lateral decubitus position only
   C. with the patient in the right lateral decubitus position only
   D. with the patient in the erect position only
   E. none of the above

E is correct.
No gallbladder examination should be performed using only one position, if possible. Multiple views allow for a more thorough and accurate examination.

2.027 To evaluate the patency of the cystic duct, it is possible to:
- A. view it directly by imaging the duct
- B. locate the valves of Heister in the duct
- C. administer cholecystokinin (CCK) to the patient, watching for contraction of the gallbladder
- D. assume patency if the gallbladder fails to contract after administration of CCK.

C is correct.
Gallbladder contraction is stimulated by CCK. If the gallbladder contracts after administration of this drug, this is strong evidence for patency of the cystic duct. Research studies have shown that the converse is not always true, however; failure of contraction is not specific.

2.028 When the gallbladder is in a distended state, the:
- A. wall should measure 6 mm in thickness
- B. wall should measure 7 mm in thickness
- C. wall should be < 5 mm in thickness
- D. wall should be approximately 10 mm in thickness

C is correct.
Some researchers state that the normal gallbladder wall is never > 3 mm in thickness.

2.029 The gallbladder may be distended in:
- A. patients who have consumed a fatty meal
- B. bedridden patients with chronic illnesses
- C. diabetic patients
- D. patients taking cholinergic drugs
- E. Courvoisier gallbladder
- F. B, C and E
- G. all of the above

F is correct.
These are conditions that may cause atonicity of the gallbladder.

Hepatobiliary pathology

2.030 When the gallbladder cannot be visualized in the right upper quadrant, the sonographer should consider:
- A. gallbladder agenesis
- B. an ectopic gallbladder located posterior to the lateral segment of the left lobe of the liver
- C. an ectopic gallbladder located intrahepatically
- D. a contracted gallbladder
- E. A and B
- F. A and C
- G. all of the above

E is correct.
Agenesis of the gallbladder is a rare congenital anomaly. Ectopic gallbladders may originate from abnormal migration of the gallbladder bud. The most common location is under the left hepatic lobe, followed by an intrahepatic gallbladder. This is defined as a gallbladder in the right upper quadrant that is completely surrounded by hepatic tissue. This can be seen easily in the right upper quadrant. A contracted gallbladder, although more difficult to visualize, may be located in the right upper quadrant.

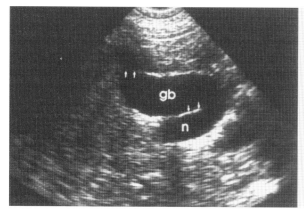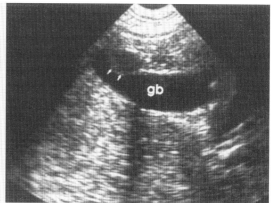

Use the above scan to answer question 2.031.

2.031 The gallbladder imaged in the sonogram represents a:
  A. bicameral gallbladder
  B. a gallbladder with a 'Phrygian cap'
  C. a double gallbladder
  D. a multiseptate gallbladder

B is correct.
A 'Phrygian cap' is a fold in the gallbladder wall near the fundus. A bicameral gallbladder is partitioned into two chambers – fundal and ductal. Double and multiseptate gallbladders are rare congenital anomalies.

2.032 A predisposition for gallstones occurs in:
  A. obese patients
  B. women more than men
  C. patients with biliary infections
  D. patients with alcoholic cirrhosis
  E. all of the above

E is correct.
Other predisposing factors include women in pregnancy or receiving estrogen, hyperlipidemia, diabetes, ileal disease and hemolytic anemias.

2.033 The finding of _____ is/are most typical of chronic cirrhosis of the liver.
  A. an enlarged hypoechoic liver
  B. multiple intrahepatic masses of variable echogenicity
  C. a small liver with increased echogenicity
  D. common bile duct dilation

C is correct.
In chronic cirrhosis, the liver parenchyma heals with scarring due to chronic injury or inflammation and undergoes diffuse fibrosis. The liver shrinks in size, becomes nodular, and demonstrates increased echogenicity and coarseness.

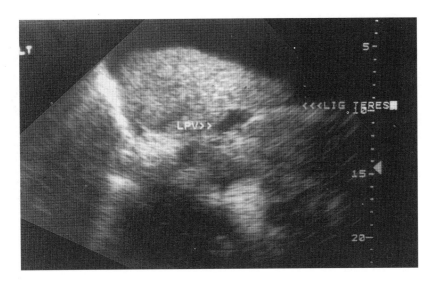

Use the above scan to answer question 2.034.

2.034 In this sonogram, what sequela of chronic cirrhosis is shown?

    A. enlarged right lobe

    B. enlarged caudate lobe

    C. benign ascites

    D. malignant ascites

C is correct.

'Benign' or transudative ascites is a feature often observed in chronic cirrhosis or congestive heart disease. The fluid is clear and may be observed to be free-flowing by positioning the patient in the decubiti positions. 'Malignant' or exudative ascites involves a thickened fluid filled with echo-producing cellular debris, proteins, etc. It may have septations and is not free-flowing. This type is characteristic of a malignant or inflammatory process.

2.035 The first location at which ascites collects in the right upper quadrant is:

    A. the porta hepatis region

    B. Morrison's pouch

    C. in the anterior subphrenic space

    D. in the lesser sac

B is correct.

Morrison's pouch, or the hepatorenal pouch, lies between the right kidney and right lobe of the liver.

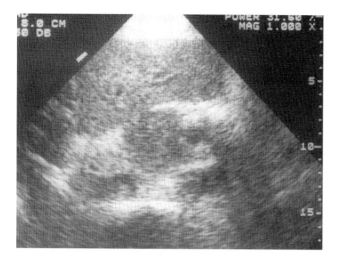

Use the above scan to answer question 2.036.

2.036 What hallmark(s) of pathology is/are identified in this scan?
- A. increased liver echogenicity – chronic cirrhosis
- B. relatively enlarged right lobe – chronic cirrhosis
- C. relatively enlarged caudate lobe – chronic cirrhosis
- D. decreased echogenicity – acute hepatitis
- E. ascites – chronic cirrhosis
- F. A and C
- G. B and C

F is correct.
The caudate lobe has its own blood supply and is the least compromised vascularly in cirrhosis. The ratio between the transverse width of the caudate lobe and the right lobe may be calculated to help in this diagnosis. According to Harbin's research, if this ratio is > 0.73, cirrhosis can be diagnosed with 99% confidence.

2.037 Cirrhosis:
- A. may have a similar appearance to fatty infiltration of the liver in the early stages
- B. causes hepatomegaly when it is advanced
- C. is reversible at the chronic stage
- D. is caused by portal hypertension

A is correct.
Both fatty infiltration and cirrhosis exhibit coarsening and an increase in liver echogenicity. The liver may still be normal-sized in early cirrhosis. Portal hypertension is a result of cirrhosis and not a cause.

2.038 Type I glycogen storage disease (von Gierke's disease) produces:
- A. a hypoechoic enlarged liver
- B. a hypoechoic shrunken liver
- C. an echogenic enlarged liver
- D. an echogenic nodular shrunken liver

C is correct.
This disease is also associated with hepatic adenomas and focal nodular hyperplasia.

2.039 Focal nodular hyperplasia of the liver:
- A. is associated with the use of oral contraceptives
- B. may be confused with metastatic disease
- C. is characterized by a central scar from which fibrous septations radiate
- D. is usually highly echogenic
- E. is most frequently located in the porta hepatis region
- F. A and B
- G. A, B and C
- H. C and D

G is correct.
Focal nodular hyperplasia is usually hypoechoic compared with normal liver tissue and is most frequently located near the liver periphery.

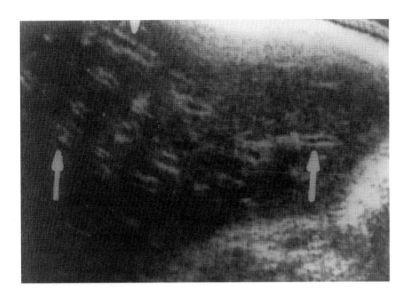

Use the above scan to answer question 2.040.

2.040 The patient, a 40-year-old man, presented with jaundice, nausea and vomiting. This sonogram was taken of the right upper quadrant. The MOST likely differential diagnosis is:
    A. acute cholecystitis
    B. pancreatitis
    C. acute hepatitis
    D. cirrhosis
    E. metastatic disease

C is correct.
In acute hepatitis, the portal venous radicals appear bright against a hypoechoic parenchymal background.

2.041 Congenital liver cysts arise from:
    A. infection from echinococcal worms
    B. adult polycystic liver disease
    C. infection from amoebic organisms
    D. developmental defects in the formation of the biliary ducts

D is correct.
'Congenital' indicates presence at birth.

2.042 The 'water-lily sign' visualized in the liver is pathognomonic for:
    A. amoebic abscesses
    B. echinococcal disease
    C. pyogenic abscesses
    D. metastatic lesions
    E. polycystic disease of the liver

B is correct.
This sign occurs when a membrane separates from the outer pericyst in echinococcal disease. The etiology of this disease (also known as hydatid disease) is a parasitic worm that is spread from the feces of dogs, cattle, etc. to humans, where it enters the gastrointestinal tract. From there, it eventually lodges in the capillaries of both the systemic and portal systems. In the liver, the larvae encyst and may reach massive size. On occasion, they form cysts within cysts (daughter cysts).

2.043 A 43-year-old woman presented clinically with fever, pain, nausea and vomiting. Her liver function tests were elevated and blood tests revealed leukocytosis. Her sonogram revealed bright echogenic foci in the liver. The MOST likely differential diagnosis is:
    A. polycystic liver disease
    B. chronic cirrhosis
    C. pyogenic bacterial abscess
    D. metastases from the gastrointestinal tract
    E. echinococcal disease

C is correct.
Abscesses in the liver are most often caused by *Escherichia coli*, *Clostridium*, or *Bacteroides*. Bright echogenic foci with 'dirty' shadowing may represent the gas produced by these organisms. Ultrasound is also helpful in guiding puncture of an abscess for drainage.

2.044 A disease which causes an intense fibrotic response in the liver and obstruction of the portal system is:
    A. lipodystrophy
    B. hepatitis
    C. echinococcal disease
    D. schistosomiasis
    E. hepatoma

D is correct.
Schistosomiasis occurs when the body is infected by a worm which invades the colonic mucosa. Ova from this worm may invade the portal venous system. The liver appears normal in size or small with regions of increased echogenicity. Dense echogenic bands are seen next to the portal veins.

2.045 In Budd–Chiari syndrome:
    A. there is obstruction to portal venous flow
    B. there is obstruction to hepatic venous flow
    C. the IVC is always occluded
    D. the liver becomes smaller
    E. there may be thrombosis in the hepatic veins
    F. A and C
    G. B and E
    H. A, C and D

G is correct.
In Budd–Chiari syndrome, the liver is enlarged and tender. There may be occlusion of the IVC and/or major hepatic veins and/or smaller centrilobular veins. The etiology of this syndrome may be unknown; however, it is associated with hypercoagulable states, collagen–vascular diseases, oral contraceptives, hepatic tumors and radiation therapy.

2.046 In Budd–Chiari syndrome, in a state of partial occlusion, vascular Doppler should demonstrate:
    A. hepatofugal flow in the right portal vein
    B. hepatopetal flow in the right portal vein
    C. no flow in the right portal vein
    D. no flow in the left portal vein

A is correct.
When a portal vein is affected by Budd–Chiari syndrome, blood flows away from the liver (hepatofugally); in unaffected vessels, blood flows in the usual direction (hepatopetally).

2.047 Portal hypertension is often accompanied by:
    A. recanalization of the ligamentum teres (umbilical vein)
    B. recanalization of the ligamentum venosum (ductus venosus)
    C. splenomegaly
    D. esophageal varices
    E. A, C and D
    F. all of the above

E is correct.
These sequelae are a result of hepatofugal blood flow in the portal system.

2.048 After liver transplantation, the MOST serious complication in the early post-transplant period is:
    A. ascites
    B. hepatic artery thrombosis
    C. formation of calcifications in the liver
    D. hepatic vein thrombosis

B is correct.
The incidence of thrombosis is described as 3–12% in adults and 11–42% in children. Duplex and color Doppler evaluation of the hepatic artery can assess patency of the vessel.

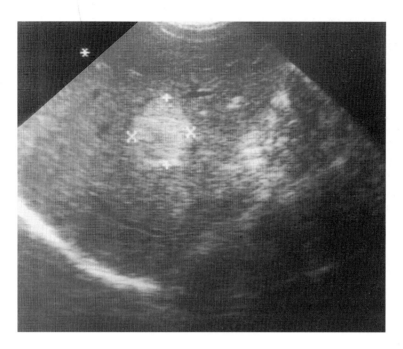

Use the above scan to answer question 2.049.

2.049 The common hepatic benign tumor visualized on this sonogram is MOST likely:
    A. an adenocarcinoma
    B. a cavernous hemangioma
    C. a primary hepatoma
    D. a lymphoma
    E. a metastasis from the gastrointestinal tract

B is correct.
These vascular tumors, found most often in women, are usually homogeneous, well-marginated and hyperechoic, and may display posterior enhancement. Patients are usually asymptomatic. Technically, they are arteriovenous malformations and not true neoplasms.

2.050 A malignant tumor associated with cirrhosis and chronic hepatitis B is:
    A. lipoma
    B. hepatocellular carcinoma
    C. lymphoma
    D. hemangioma
    E. liver abscess

B is correct.
Patients often present with a palpable mass, rapid liver enlargement and a low fever. Often, alpha-fetoprotein (AFP) levels in the blood are elevated. Liver function deteriorates more rapidly than would be expected from the underlying cirrhosis or chronic hepatitis B alone.

2.051 Ultrasonographically, hepatocellular carcinoma may appear as:
    A. several discrete hypoechoic masses in the liver
    B. echogenic discrete masses in the liver
    C. complex masses with indistinguishable borders
    D. diffuse infiltrative tumors throughout the liver
    E. tumors undergoing liquefaction necrosis
    F. all of the above

F is correct.
The appearances of these tumors are variable, depending on the age of the tumor. Research has shown that these tumors evolve with time from small hypoechoic or isoechoic masses to large hyperechoic complex masses.

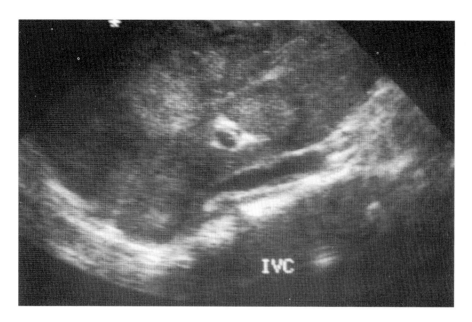

Use the above scan to answer question 2.052.

2.052 The patient presented with hepatomegaly, and elevated levels of AST (SGOT), ALT (SGPT) and alpha-fetoprotein. The MOST likely differential diagnosis for this sonogram of the right upper quadrant is:

    A. hemangioma
    B. hepatocellular carcinoma
    C. metastasis from the gastrointestinal tract
    D. hepatic hematoma
    E. lymphoma

C is correct.
This sonogram has the characteristic 'bull's-eye' or 'target' signs that metastases from the gastrointestinal tract may demonstrate. However, metastases may present with a wide variety of appearances, reflecting the spectrum of tumor types. For example, echogenic masses often arise from metastatic cancer of the colon whereas cystic necrosis is associated with leiomyosarcomas and hypoechoic masses with lymphomas.

2.053 Which of the following is a TRUE description of the evolution of a hematoma in the liver?

    A. anechoic mass, complex mass, anechoic mass
    B. complex mass, anechoic mass, calcified mass
    C. septated echogenic mass, calcified mass
    D. anechoic mass, target sign, anechoic mass

A is correct.
The appearance of a hematoma depends on the age of the bleed. Initially, fresh blood in liquid form appears anechoic. As the clotting process occurs, a hematoma gives a more complex appearance; during resolution, a seroma is formed which again exhibits an anechoic cystic appearance.

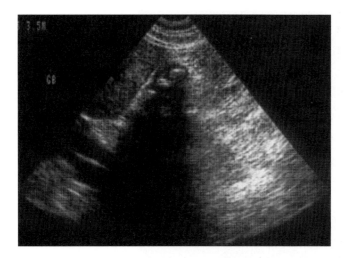

Use the above scan to answer question 2.054.

2.054 This sonogram of the right upper quadrant demonstrates the characteristic:
    A. 'bull's-eye' sign
    B. 'WES' sign
    C. 'target' sign
    D. 'too many tubes' sign

B is correct.
'WES' stands for 'wall, echo and shadow', representing the anterior wall of a contracted gallbladder, echogenic calculi, and posterior acoustic shadowing. This sign is usually seen in chronic cholecystitis.

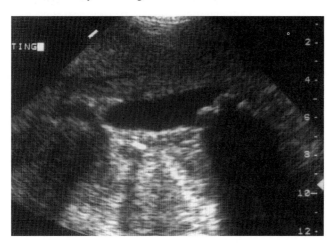

Use the above scan to answer question 2.055.

2.055 Gallstones are imaged in this sonogram in the:
    A. neck of the gallbladder
    B. body of the gallbladder
    C. cystic duct
    D. fundus

D is correct.
This patient had rolling stones. Gallstones originally imaged in the body of the gallbladder rolled to the fundus when the patient sat up. True gallstones are gravity-dependent and move when the patient changes position. This is an important diagnostic criterion for gallstones because polyps and other mural lesions are fixed in position.

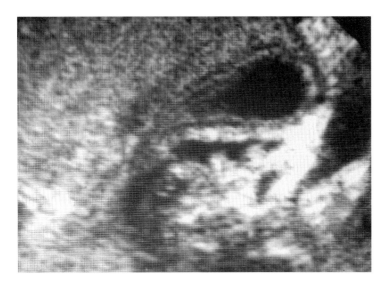

Use the above scan to answer question 2.056.

2.056 The patient presented with right upper quadrant tenderness, fever, nausea and vomiting. The MOST likely diagnosis on the basis of this sonogram is:
    A. calculous cholecystitis
    B. gallbladder carcinoma
    C. acalculous cholecystitis
    D. cholelithiasis

C is correct.
Acalculous cholecystitis has the same signs and symptoms as calculous cholecystitis. It shows a male predominance and is influenced by predisposing factors such as congenital biliary malformations, vascular disorders, trauma, extensive burns and dehydration, among other factors. In this scan, posterior to the gallbladder is a fluid-filled duodenum.

2.057 In acute cholecystitis:
    A. an occluded cystic duct may be directly visualized sonographically
    B. Murphy's sign is detected when scanning directly over the gallbladder
    C. the wall of the gallbladder should exceed 5 mm in thickness
    D. there may be a 'halo' sign around the gallbladder
    E. there is always complete contraction of the gallbladder
    F. A and B
    G. B and C
    H. B, C and D

H is correct.
Murphy's sign is detected when maximum tenderness is felt by the patient when the probe is passed directly over the gallbladder. The 'halo' represents subserosal edema around the wall. Pericholecystic fluid may also be present.

2.058 The MOST common cause of obstructive jaundice is:
    A. cholelithiasis
    B. choledocholithiasis
    C. acalculous cholecystitis
    D. cholecystitis
    E. occlusion of the IVC

B is correct.
Other symptoms of obstruction of the common bile duct include right upper quadrant colicky pain radiating to the right scapula and progressive jaundice.

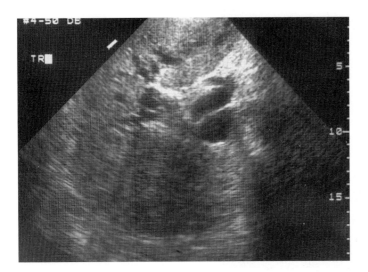

Use the above scan to answer question 2.059.

2.059 What sequela of obstruction of the common bile duct is seen in this sonogram?
    A. prominent portal radicals
    B. decreased through transmission in the liver parenchyma
    C. dilated intrahepatic biliary ducts
    D. cholecystitis

C is correct.
Biliary ducts are usually not visualized unless they enlarge due to obstruction at a lower level. They appear as anechoic tubular structures and follow a winding course adjacent to the anechoic tubular portal veins.

2.060 A dilated thick-walled gallbladder and ductal obstruction due to lymphadenopathy are characteristic of:
    A. hepatic abscesses
    B. hepatocellular carcinoma
    C. AIDS
    D. adenomyomatosis

C is correct.
AIDS patients may also demonstrate hepatic parenchymal abnormalities, including hyperechogenicity, granulomas and hepatomegaly.

2.061 When there is biliary duct dilatation without an obstructive etiology, this may represent:
    A. adenocarcinoma of the pancreas head
    B. Caroli's disease
    C. Budd–Chiari syndrome
    D. metastases from the gastrointestinal tract
    E. AIDS

B is correct.
Caroli's disease is a developmental congenital abnormality of the bile ducts. This results in ectasia (widening) of the bile ducts, leading to bile stasis and the formation of calculi. The disease may also be accompanied by a chole-dochal cyst and congenital hepatic fibrosis.

2.062 On visualization of a polypoid lesion in the gallbladder that does not demonstrate acoustic shadowing, which of the following diagnoses should be considered?
    A. cholecystitis
    B. cholangitis
    C. cholelithiasis with a cholesterol stone
    D. gallbladder carcinoma

D is correct.
Gallbladder carcinoma, the most frequent cancer of the biliary system, may demonstrate a variety of ultrasound appearances: a polypoid lesion with irregular borders; irregular thickening of the gallbladder wall; a solid mass filling the lumen of the gallbladder; or a mass infiltrating the wall of the gallbladder. It has a high association with cholelithiasis and chronic cholecystitis.

Normal pancreas

2.063 The optimal patient preparation and positioning for a pancreatic sonogram is:
   A. patient NPO for 6–8 h and in RLD position
   B. patient postprandial and in LLD position
   C. patient NPO for 6–8 h and in supine position
   D. patient NPO for 6–8 h and in prone position

C is correct.
Fasting before a pancreatic sonogram lessens bowel gas interference with the sonic beam, and gas shadowing from solid contents of the stomach, which lies anterior to the pancreas. Sipping water through a straw to fill the stomach with fluid provides a sonic window.

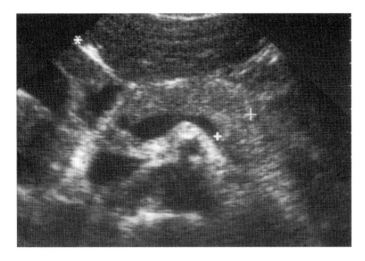

Use the above scan to answer questions 2.064 – 2.068.

2.064 In this sonogram of the pancreas, which vessel is seen in long axis directly posterior to the pancreas?
   A. superior mesenteric vein
   B. splenic vein
   C. superior mesenteric artery
   D. right portal vein

B is correct.
The splenic vein originates from 5 or 6 veins in the splenic hilus, and courses posterior to the body and tail of the pancreas. It unites with the superior mesenteric vein to form the main portal vein.

2.065 In this sonogram, what is being measured by the calipers?
   A. uncinate process
   B. spleen
   C. body of pancreas
   D. tail of pancreas
   E. head of the pancreas

D is correct.
In a normal patient, the tail of the pancreas usually measures up to 2.8 cm

2.066 In this sonogram, what structure may be identified immediately to the right and lateral to the head of the pancreas?
   A. common bile duct
   B. common hepatic duct
   C. descending duodenum
   D. third portion of the duodenum
   E. gallbladder

C is correct.
In this sonogram, the duodenum appears to be filled with fluid, which is helpful in delineating the contour of the head. The C-loop of the duodenum has three portions: superior or first portion; descending or second portion; and bottom of the loop or third portion, also called the transverse or horizontal portion. The fourth and final part of the duodenum, distal to the C-loop, ascends into the left upper quadrant and ends at the ligament of Treitz.

2.067 In this sonogram, what is used as a sonic window to aid visualization of the pancreas?
- A. a water-filled stomach
- B. positioning the patient in the right lateral decubitus position
- C. the lateral segment of the left lobe of liver
- D. the medial segment of the left lobe of liver

C is correct.

The larger this segment of the liver, the better it is to visualize the pancreas posterior to it. The sinusoids of the liver are filled with blood, thus facilitating the ultrasonic beam. Filling the stomach with water is another good technique for delineating the pancreas. However, this technique was not used in this sonogram.

2.068 In this sonogram, the common bile duct:
- A. is seen in long axis in the body of the pancreas
- B. is seen uniting with the pancreatic duct in the head of the pancreas
- C. is seen in short axis in the head of the pancreas
- D. is seen posterior to the head of the pancreas

C is correct.

The common bile duct appears as an anechoic circle in the posterior portion of the head of the pancreas.

2.069 In sagittal section:
- A. the head of the pancreas is seen anterior to the aorta
- B. the body of the pancreas is seen anterior to the aorta
- C. the head of the pancreas is seen posterior to the IVC
- D. the body of the pancreas is seen posterior to the aorta
- E. the uncinate process is never seen

B is correct.

The head and uncinate process of the pancreas are seen anterior to the IVC.

2.070 The smallest portion of the pancreas in anterior–posterior diameter is the:
- A. head
- B. body
- C. neck
- D. tail
- E. uncinate process

C is correct.

The neck of the gland measures approximately 10 mm.

Pancreatic pathology

2.071 With the aging process, the pancreas:
- A. increases in size and becomes more echogenic
- B. increases in size and has a constant echogenicity
- C. decreases in size and becomes hypoechoic
- D. decreases in size and becomes more echogenic

D is correct.

After 60 years of age, studies have revealed that there is moderate-to-severe fat deposition in the acinar cells of the pancreas. This results in the pancreas appearing more echogenic in older patients. It also decreases in size with advancing age.

2.072 The MOST common malignant pancreatic neoplasm is:

    A. adenoma
    B. lymphoma
    C. islet cell tumors
    D. cystadenocarcinomas
    E. adenocarcinoma

E is correct.
Adenocarcinoma is most commonly found in middle-aged men. Patients present with epigastric pain, anorexia, nausea, vomiting and, possibly, obstructive jaundice.

2.073 The phrase 'small tumors that are hypo- or isoechoic to pancreatic tissue' MOST closely describes:

    A. islet cell tumors
    B. lymphomas
    C. adenocarcinomas
    D. metastases
    E. pancreatic pseudocysts

A is correct.
Because of their small size and their hypo- or isoechogenicity to the rest of the pancreas, they are difficult to detect sonographically. They may be functionally active, thus giving a clinical hint to their presence. The most common islet cell tumor is an insulinoma, which can be either benign or malignant. Islet cell tumors are more common in the body and tail regions whereas acinar or exocrine tumors are more common in the head of the pancreas.

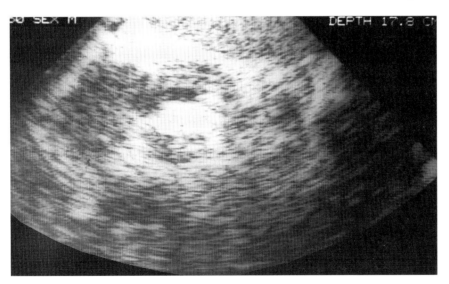

Use the above scan to answer question 2.074.

2.074 A 62-year-old man presented with nausea and vomiting, and jaundice. This upper abdominal sonogram was taken of the patient and MOST likely depicts:

    A. a complex mass in the body of the pancreas –
       adenocarcinoma
    B. a cystic mass in the head of the pancreas –
       cystadenocarcinoma
    C. a hypoechoic mass in the tail of the pancreas –
       lymphoma
    D. a solid mass in the head of the pancreas –
       adenocarcinoma

D is correct.
Adenocarcinoma usually presents as a solid focal enlargement of the head of the pancreas. It is usually hypoechoic in relation to the rest of the pancreatic tissue and has poor transonicity.

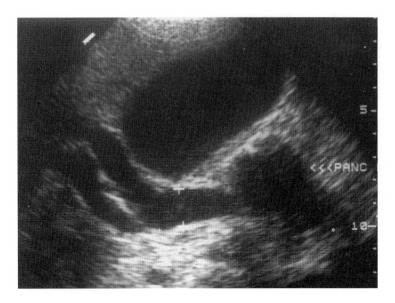

Use the above scan to answer question 2.075.

2.075 What is seen in this sonogram that is a sequela to a mass in the head of the pancreas?
    A. dilated intrahepatic duct dilatation and enlarged gallbladder
    B. dilated common bile duct and enlarged gallbladder
    C. dilated duct of Wirsung and dilated common duct
    D. gallstones with shadowing

B is correct.
A and C may also result, but are not seen on this particular sonogram. A palpable non-tender gallbladder is referred to as a Courvoisier gallbladder.

2.076 Using ultrasound, the duct of Wirsung:
    A. measures 5 mm and is usually seen in the pancreatic head
    B. measures 2 mm and is usually seen in the pancreatic body
    C. measures 1 mm and cannot be seen unless it is dilated
    D. measures 10 mm and is usually seen in the pancreatic body

B is correct.
Portions of the duct are usually seen in the body region. They are tubular and appear as an anechoic lumen bordered by echogenic lines.

2.077 In the course of adenocarcinoma of the pancreas, the 'cuff sign' is recognized when:
    A. there is thickening of the gallbladder wall
    B. there is an increase in size of the pancreas
    C. there is portal hypertension diagnosed by Doppler
    D. there is prominent thickening around the superior mesenteric artery caused by local tumor invasion

D is correct.
If this sign is discovered, usually the pancreatic tumor is non-resectable by surgery.

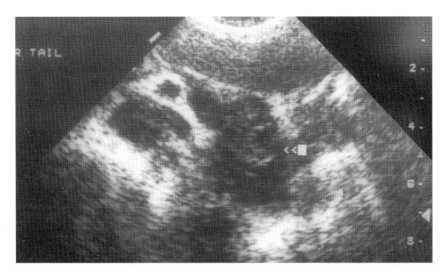

Use the above scan to answer question 2.078.

2.078 An asymptomatic 56-year-old man took this screening upper abdominal sonogram as part of a yearly physical examination. What pathology is identified in this sonogram?
    A. pancreatic pseudocyst in the tail of the pancreas
    B. a neoplasm in the tail of the pancreas
    C. a neoplasm in the body of the pancreas
    D. a neoplasm in the stomach
    E. dilated splenic flexure

B is correct.
Neoplasms in this region are the latest to present with symptoms as they do not cause obstruction of the biliary system.

2.079 Which one of the following is TRUE of mucinous cystadenomas and adenocarcinomas of the pancreas?
    A. they are mainly found in their benign form (adenoma)
    B. they are found more frequently in the head region of the pancreas
    C. the cysts are usually unilocular and > 2 cm
    D. they are poorly marginated and have mixed echogenicity

C is correct.
Mucinous cyst tumors are potentially malignant tumors and 60% are located in the tail region. Microcystic neoplasms are more often benign, and consist of multiple tiny cysts with fibrous walls that are responsible for their echogenic appearance.

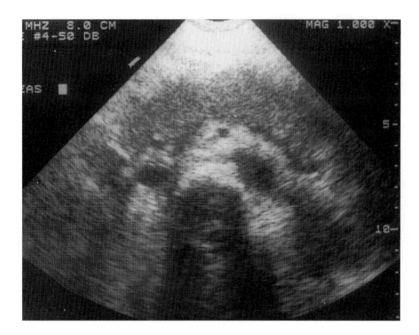

Use the above scan to answer question 2.080.

2.080 This is a sonogram of a 24-year-old man with a history of alcohol abuse, who presented with intense epigastric pain, nausea and vomiting. Blood tests revealed elevated amylase and lipase levels. The MOST likely diagnosis is:
    A. chronic pancreatitis
    B. pancreatic pseudocyst in the head region
    C. acute pancreatitis
    D. chronic pancreatitis
    E. pancreatic neoplasm

C is correct.
Acute pancreatitis appears sonographically as either a normal or enlarged hypoechoic gland. In this sonogram, the pancreas appears puffy, hypoechoic to the liver and diffusely enlarged. This is associated with biliary tract disease (gallstones) and alcoholism.

2.081 Pancreatic pseudocysts are a common sequela of:
    A. chronic pancreatitis
    B. chronic cholecystitis
    C. acute pancreatitis
    D. adenocarcinoma of the pancreas

C is correct.
Pseudocysts occur in 10–50% of patients with acute pancreatitis. They are collections of fluid and debris resulting from tissue digested by pancreatic juice. Their walls are usually thick and composed of fibrous tissue, unlike true cysts, which are lined by epithelium.

2.082 Which of the following represents locations of extrapancreatic pseudocysts in the order of the most common to the least common?
    A. anterior pararenal space, lesser sac, posterior pararenal space, mediastinum
    B. lesser sac, anterior pararenal space, posterior pararenal space, mediastinum
    C. greater sac, lesser sac, anterior pararenal space, posterior pararenal space
    D. posterior pararenal space, anterior pararenal space, lesser sac, small bowel mesentery

B is correct.
Rarely, a pseudocyst may extend into the mediastinum through the aortic or esophageal hiatus.

2.083 Which of the following describes a typical sonographic appearance of a pseudocyst?

    A. complex mass in the head of the pancreas with poor through transmission

    B. multiple cystic masses throughout the pancreas with good through transmission

    C. cystic mass in the tail region with good through transmission

    D. solid mass in the body of the pancreas with good through transmission

C is correct.

Pseudocysts may be situated within or adjacent to any region of the pancreas, but are found particularly in the tail. They vary in size and are usually single cystic masses displaying good transonicity.

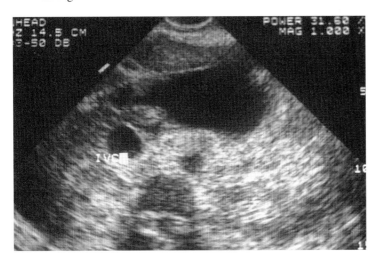

Use the above scan to answer question 2.084.

2.084 What pathology is imaged in this sonogram?

    A. water-filled stomach

    B. Courvoisier gallbladder

    C. pancreatic pseudocyst

    D. pancreatic phlegmon

    E. microcystic adenocarcinoma

C is correct.

Although this cystic mass has the contour of a gallbladder, do not be fooled. Note its position in relation to the pancreas head and body, and the IVC.

2.085 Long-standing chronic pancreatitis usually appears sonographically as:

    A. a shrunken echogenic gland with calcifications

    B. an enlarged echogenic gland with calcifications

    C. a hypoechoic enlarged gland without calcifications

    D. a shrunken hypoechoic gland with calcifications

A is correct.

As pancreatitis progresses, there is destruction and atrophy of the acini, an increase of fibrous tissue, chronic inflammatory infiltration and formation of calcifications. It is associated with alcoholism and biliary tract disease, and is more common in men than in women.

2.086 In acute pancreatitis, an inflammatory process that spreads to soft tissues around the pancreas to cause edema and swelling is:

    A. a pancreatic pseudocyst

    B. a phlegmon

    C. a hematoma

    D. an abscess

    E. a region of liquefaction necrosis

B is correct.

A phlegmon occurs in around 20% of patients with acute pancreatitis. It appears to be hypoechoic with good through transmission.

2.087 An etiology for a very echogenic pancreas is:
   A. pancreatic pseudocyst
   B. acute pancreatitis
   C. phlegmon
   D. hemorrhagic pancreatitis
   E. cystic fibrosis

E is correct.
In cystic fibrosis, there is secretion of abnormally thick mucus, which causes obstruction of the pancreatic ductal system. The ducts undergo cystic degeneration and ultimately fibrosis.

Normal kidney

2.088 Which of the following is TRUE with regard to echogenicity relationships in the kidney?
   A. medulla > cortex > renal sinus
   B. renal sinus > cortex > medulla
   C. cortex > medulla > renal sinus
   D. cortex < medulla < renal sinus

B is correct.
The echo intensity of the adult renal sinus is mainly due to adipose tissue in the hilar region. The cortex displays moderate echogenicity and the medullary pyramids usually appear relatively hypoechoic.

2.089 In the adult, which of the following would be considered an enlarged kidney?
   A. 10–12 cm in length; 5–6 cm in transverse; 3–4 cm in AP
   B. 8–10 cm in length; 5–6 cm in transverse; 3–4 cm in AP
   C. 12–14 cm in length; 5–6 cm in transverse; 5–6 cm in AP
   D. 7–8 cm in length; 4–5 cm in transverse; 4–5 cm in AP

C is correct.
Answer A gives what is considered by most to be normal dimensions, which vary with age, gender and body habitus. Often, renal enlargement is first noted in the AP (anterior–posterior) dimension with 'rounding' of the kidney.

2.090 The optimal technique for scanning the right kidney is:
   A. supine, intercostally and in deep inspiration
   B. supine, subcostally and in deep inspiration
   C. in left lateral decubitus, subcostally and in suspended respiration
   D. all of the above

D is correct.
Various approaches to scanning may be successful, depending on body habitus and the position of the kidney in the patient.

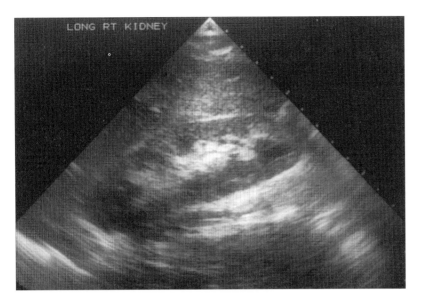

LONG RT KIDNEY

Use the above scan to answer questions 2.091—2.093.

2.091 In this sonogram of the kidney, which pole is located MOST posteriorly in the body?
  A. lower pole
  B. upper pole
  C. midpole
  D. all poles are equidistant from the posterior of the body

B is correct.
The upper poles are oriented relatively posterior to the rest of the kidney, which is parallel to the long axis of the psoas muscle.

2.092 In this sonogram, what is seen dipping between the renal medullary pyramids?
  A. columns of Bertin
  B. renal capsule
  C. renal pelvis
  D. arcuate vessels

A is correct.
The columns of Bertin are composed of renal cortex located between the pyramids. Occasionally, a column may hypertrophy and mimic a renal mass.

2.093 In this sonogram, the MOST hyperechoic portion is the:
  A. medullary pyramids
  B. renal sinus
  C. cortex
  D. columns of Bertin

B is correct.
The echo intensity of the sinus is caused by hilar adipose tissue, and the presence of blood vessels and the collecting system.

2.094 Of the following, the easiest renal vessel(s) to identify using B scanning is/are:
  A. the main renal artery
  B. lobar arteries
  C. segmental arteries
  D. arcuate arteries

A is correct.
This is the largest renal vessel in anatomical terms. However, with Doppler, all of the arteries can be distinguished by their characteristic spectral analysis.

Renal pathology

2.095 The MOST common renal congenital anomaly is:
  A. cross-fused ectopia
  B. duplicated collecting system
  C. pelvic kidney
  D. thoracic kidney

B is correct.
Found more frequently in women, duplication of the collecting system is a common congenital anomaly. Sonographically, it can be identified on visualization of a cortical separation between the hyperechoic renal sinus echoes.

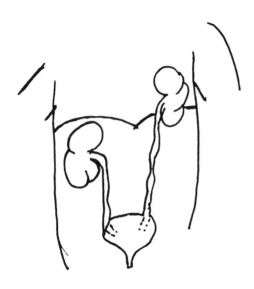

Use the above diagram to answer question 2.096.

2.096 This diagram depicts which renal congenital anomaly?
  A. cross-fused ectopia
  B. intrathoracic kidney
  C. ptotic kidney
  D. pelvic kidney

B is correct.
Associated with delayed closure of the thoracic cavity, an intrathoracic kidney is a rare occurrence. It is more commonly found on the left side.

2.097 In cross-fused ectopia, the sonographic appearance is MOST likely to appear as:
  A. an elongated kidney found only on one side of the body
  B. two kidneys joined at their poles by an isthmus of fibrous tissue
  C. a small underdeveloped kidney
  D. a kidney located in the pelvis

A is correct.
Answer B describes a horseshoe kidney, C describes hypoplasia of the kidney and D is a pelvic kidney.

2.098 A pelvic kidney:
  A. demonstrates respiratory excursions
  B. demonstrates peristalsis
  C. may or may not be functional
  D. is always completely normal anatomically

C is correct.
Pelvic kidneys occur when a kidney fails to ascend during embryological development.

2.099 Horseshoe kidneys are:
   A. normally located in the pelvis
   B. fused together on one side of the body
   C. joined by an isthmus that courses anterior to the
      great vessels
   D. usually fused by their upper poles

C is correct.
Horseshoe kidneys are often discovered when patients are referred to ultrasound for evaluation of a pulsatile mass, as the isthmus courses anterior to the aorta. Fusion occurs at the lower poles in 90% of cases.

2.100 If a sonographer suspects the presence of a pelvic kidney, the FIRST thing to do is:
   A. alert the physician
   B. look in both renal fossae for the presence of kidneys
   C. perform a spectral analysis of the 'mass'
   D. refer the patient for a renal nuclear scan to determine
      renal function

B is correct.
All of the other responses are valid, but the first thing to do is to search in both renal fossae for the presence of normal kidneys. Supernumerary kidneys are **extremely** rare!

2.101 Fetal lobulations:
   A. are congenital anomalies
   B. only occur in the right kidney
   C. may be confused with a solid renal mass
   D. are often more prominent in the left kidney
   E. A and C
   F. C and D

F is correct.
Renal lobulations are a normal stage in fetal embryological development. Occasionally, a remnant of this fetal stage remains after birth. The fetal 'hump' is most commonly noted in the lateral aspect of the left kidney.

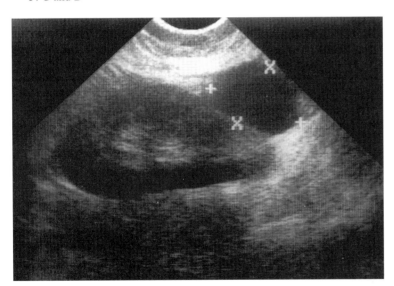

Use the above scan to answer question 2.102.

2.102 With regard to this sonogram, which criteria and diagnosis match?
   A. poor through transmission – solid mass
   B. posterior enhancement – a simple renal cyst
   C. posterior enhancement, rounded contour,
      anechoic – simple renal cyst
   D. rounded contour – hemorrhagic cyst

C is correct.
To be classified as a **simple** cyst anywhere in the body, a mass must display an anechoic interior, smooth walls, rounded contour and posterior enhancement.

2.103 Multicystic dysplastic kidney disease differs from infantile polycystic kidney disease because the former:
   A. displays a kidney filled with cysts of varying sizes
   B. is inherited as an autosominal-dominant
   C. is filled with tiny cysts that give a hyperechoic appearance
   D. is usually seen unilaterally as the bilateral form is inconsistent with life
   E. A and D
   F. B and C
   G. A and B

E is correct.
Multicystic dysplastic kidney develops from complete ureteral obstruction *in utero*. Terminal tubules become cysts that do not communicate, but become joined together by small connective tissue cords. It is a non-functional kidney. The main role of ultrasound is to distinguish between multicystic dysplastic kidney and hydronephrosis.

2.104 A neonate presents sonographically with bilaterally enlarged hyperechoic kidneys. The MOST likely diagnosis is:
   A. adult polycystic kidney disease
   B. renal angiomyolipomas
   C. infantile polycystic disease
   D. staghorn calculi
   E. multicystic dysplastic kidney disease

C is correct.
Infantile polycystic kidney disease (IPKD) is inherited as an autosomal-recessive and, in its most severe form, presents as bilaterally enlarged kidneys filled with tiny echogenic cysts.

2.105 The type of IPKD associated with the LEAST renal involvement, and the MOST hepatic fibrosis and portal hypertension is:
   A. perinatal
   B. neonatal
   C. infantile
   D. juvenile

D is correct.
IPKD may be classified into four types:
perinatal: at birth, 90% of renal tubules involved, minimal liver fibrosis;
neonatal: birth to 8 months, intermediate renal and liver involvement;
infantile: up to 7 years, intermediate renal and liver involvement;
juvenile: older children, 10% of renal tubules involved, maximum hepatic fibrosis.
All types eventually develop progressive renal failure.

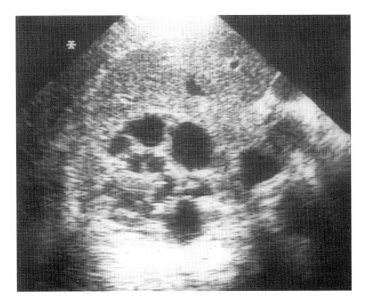

Use the above scan to answer question 2.106.

2.106 Mr A, a 40-year-old pickle-packer, presents with lumbar pain and proteinuria. This is his right renal sonogram; the left kidney had a similar appearance on ultrasound. Based on his history and this renal sonogram, the MOST likely diagnosis is:
  A. multicystic dysplastic kidney disease
  B. cystic renal neoplasm
  C. hydronephrosis
  D. adult polycystic kidney disease

D is correct.
Adult polycystic kidney disease (APKD), inherited as an autosomal-dominant, often presents in the fourth decade of life. It results in the formation of multiple cysts in both kidneys that eventually lead to renal failure. The most frequent complication is cyst hemorrhage, infection and renal calculi.

2.107 Concurrent with APKD, the MOST likely location for cysts is the:
  A. pancreas
  B. spleen
  C. liver
  D. ovaries and testes

C is correct.
Cysts in the liver are found in 25–50% of patients with APKD; 9% have cysts in the pancreas, and smaller percentages are seen in the lungs, spleen, ovaries and testes. APKD is also associated with berry aneurysms in the circle of Willis in the brain; these are prone to rupture leading to subarachnoid hemorrhages.

2.108 Parapelvic cysts:
  A. may be located anywhere in the kidney
  B. may be confused with hydronephrosis
  C. are located in the renal hilus and have no connection to the collecting system
  D. may develop from lymphatic tissue
  E. usually become hemorrhagic
  F. B and C
  G. A and B

F is correct.
Patients with parapelvic cysts are usually asymptomatic. These cysts appear as anechoic well-defined masses which only occasionally become infected or cause obstruction.

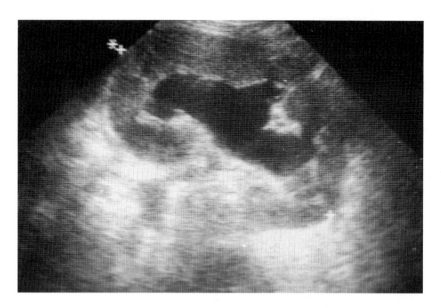

Use the above scan to answer question 2.109.

2.109 Mr H, a 65-year-old retired cat-burglar, has no family history of renal disease. He now presents with dull right lumbar pain and hematuria. Based on his history and this renal sonogram, the MOST likely diagnosis is:
    A. APKD
    B. hydronephrosis
    C. renal sinus lipomatosis
    D. renal neoplasm
    E. renal calculus

B is correct.
Hydronephrosis occurs when there is urinary dilatation of the renal pelvis and calyces. It may be the result of either intrinsic or extrinsic obstruction.

2.110 In the case of Mr H, the MOST likely cause of his problem is:
    A. renal neoplasm
    B. posterior urethral valves
    C. benign prostatic hypertrophy
    D. renal calculi

C is correct.
Benign prostatic hypertrophy, an enlargement of the prostate gland occurring in older men, is often a cause of hydronephrosis in this patient population.

2.111 Renal calculi:
    A. display good transonicity and acoustic shadowing
    B. display poor transonicity and acoustic shadowing
    C. have smooth regular contours
    D. are more common in women
    E. produce painless hematuria

B is correct.
Common in men between 30 and 55 years of age, calculi formation is influenced by hereditary factors, high concentration of stone constituents, changes in urinary pH, stasis of urine, etc. The most common symptoms are hematuria, oliguria and renal colic – very painful spasms that arise as the stone is passed down the ureter.

2.112 A renal calculus located in the upper pole of the kidney may cause:
- A. a neoplasm
- B. focal hydronephrosis
- C. formation of a renal cyst
- D. an infection
- E. A and D
- F. B and C
- G. B and D

G is correct.
If a calculus blocks a calyx in one region of the kidney, focal or localized hydronephrosis (also called caliectasis) may occur. Because of urinary stasis, there is always the possibility of infection.

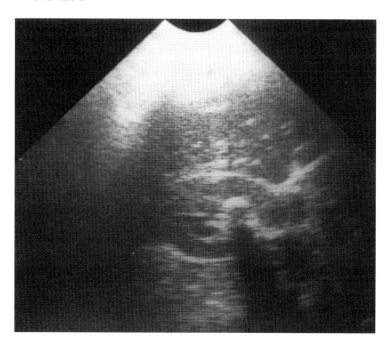

Use the above scan to answer question 2.113.

2.113 The pathology identified in this sonogram is:
- A. sinus lipomatosis
- B. staghorn calculus
- C. moderate hydronephrosis
- D. renal cell carcinoma

B is correct.
Staghorn calculus results when the entire collecting system is filled with a stone, giving an appearance resembling the antlers of a deer. Note the strong acoustic shadowing produced by the calculus.

2.114 A benign solid mass of the kidney that appears very hyperechoic is:
- A. adenocarcinoma
- B. Wilms' tumor
- C. angiomyolipoma
- D. neuroblastoma
- E. lymphoma

C is correct.
Angiomyolipomas are composed of fat, muscle and vascular tissues, hence their very echogenic appearance. They are located more commonly on the right side and are found mainly in women. Multiple angiomyolipomas occur as part of the tuberous sclerosis complex.

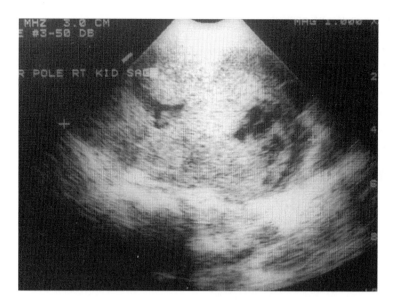

Use the above scan to answer question 2.115.

2.115 Two-year-old Willard presented with a flank mass and hypertension. This is his sonogram; what is the MOST likely diagnosis?
    A. hypernephroma
    B. lymphoma
    C. Wilms' tumor
    D. angiomyolipoma
    E. hydronephrosis

C is correct.
Wilms' tumors, or nephroblastomas, are the most common malignant renal tumor found in young children. A differential diagnosis to consider is an adrenal neuroblastoma, which may be found in the same population.

2.116 When comparing neuroblastomas to nephroblastomas, the former are usually:
    A. more homogeneous
    B. more heterogeneous
    C. more solid
    D. more sharply marginated
    E. less sharply marginated
    F. A and D
    G. B and E
    H. A and C

G is correct.
Adrenal neuroblastomas are malignant tumors also found in young children. Although these sonographic differences between tumors may have validity, remember that they are only generalizations.

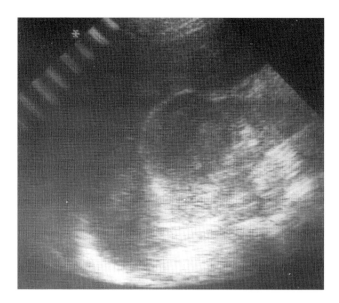

Use the above scan to answer question 2.117.

2.117 Mr M, a 61-year-old pizza-twirler, presented with
painless hematuria. After sonographic evaluation, the
MOST likely diagnosis is:
    A. lymphoma
    B. nephroblastoma
    C. hypernephroma
    D. metastatic cancer

C is correct.
Hypernephromas, or renal adenocarcinomas, are
found in the group ages 50–70 years, with a
male-to-female ratio of 3:1. They are generally
hypoechoic, producing an irregular renal contour
and distortion of the renal architecture.

2.118 When there is leukemic infiltration, the kidneys:
    A. appear enlarged with multiple anechoic nodular areas
       or are diffusely infiltrated
    B. appear shrunken with multiple anechoic nodular areas
    C. appear to have an enhanced distinction between
       cortex and medulla
    D. appear with calculi and acoustic shadowing

A is correct.
Research has shown that there is renal infiltration
in 63% of leukemias. Elevated blood pressure
and enlarged kidneys are primary symptoms of
the disease.

2.119 An enlarged kidney displaying decreased
echogenicity of the parenchyma and a pronounced back
wall is characteristic of:
    A. chronic pyelonephritis
    B. acute pyelonephritis
    C. renal abscess
    D. hydronephrosis

B is correct.
Although the most common ultrasound finding in
acute pyelonephritis is a normal examination, it
may present with renal enlargement due to
inflammation and edema. Multiple small
abscesses and necrosis are responsible for the
changes in echogenicity of the parenchyma. The
back-wall echo appears stronger than that of a
normal kidney because of the increased fluid
content of the kidney. Chronic pyelonephritis
appears sonographically as a shrunken kidney
with increased echoes due to scarring and
fibrosis.

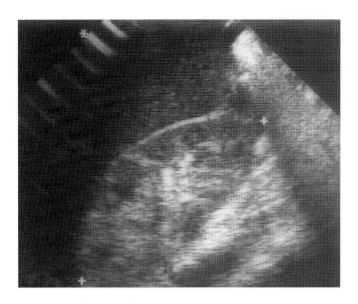

Use the above scan to answer question 2.120.

2.120 Mrs O, a diabetic, presented with fever, chills and flank pain. This is the sonogram of her right kidney. What is the MOST likely diagnosis?
  A. adenocarcinoma
  B. chronic atrophic pyelonephritis
  C. renal fungus ball
  D. acute focal bacterial nephritis

D is correct.
Acute focal bacterial nephritis, or lobar nephronia, is an inflammation of the kidney without drainable pus. It is usually caused by gram-negative bacteria (e.g. *Escherichia coli*) that ascend through ureteral reflux. Female diabetics represent most of the population affected by this infection. Its characteristic sonographic appearance consists of a poorly defined hypoechoic mass, and a loss of definition between cortex and medulla. If the mass becomes more sonolucent, an abscess must be considered. Choice A is a possibility based on ultrasound appearance alone. Regarding choice C, renal fungus balls appear as echogenic non-shadowing masses in the collecting system.

2.121 Spectral analysis of the kidneys by Doppler is usually conducted to:
  A. detect hydronephrosis
  B. detect blood flow in the venous system
  C. evaluate possible stenoses in the renal artery and its branches
  D. search for congenital anomalies

C is correct.
Stenosis in the renal arteries is an important secondary source of hypertension. Doppler studies examine flow in the main renal artery, segmental branches, interlobar branches and arcuate arteries. The resistance index (RI) may be calculated at each level as RI = (peak systolic shift − minimum systolic shift)/ peak systolic shift

2.122 If a renal artery has a partial obstruction:
    A. the blood flow velocity is decreased after the
       obstruction
    B. the blood flow velocity is increased after the
       obstruction
    C. there is no change in blood flow velocity
    D. there is no flow at all due to the obstruction

B is correct.
A narrowing in the diameter of a vessel always causes an increase in velocity of a liquid.

2.123 Color Doppler sonography and spectral analysis of a transplanted kidney can provide information on:
    A. resistance indices of the renal arteries
    B. possible renal vein thrombosis
    C. arteriovenous fissures
    D. all of the above

D is correct.
The high resistance indices found in a transplanted kidney may have many causes: acute or chronic rejection; acute tubular necrosis; infection; or cyclosporin A toxicity (a drug given to suppress the immune system). Color is helpful in locating vessels, possible stenoses or thromboses and arteriovenous fissures.

2.124 Acute renal transplant rejection is characterized by:
    A. a marked increase in renal size, specifically,
       anteroposterior ≥ transverse measurement
    B. a marked decrease in renal size
    C. a resistance index (RI) > 0.90
    D. increased echogenicity of medullary pyramids
    E. A and C
    F. B and D
    G. A, C and D

E is correct.
Acute rejection is characterized by one or more of the following signs: swelling or enlargement of the kidney; conspicuous and enlarged pyramids; decreased renal sinus fat density; and infundibular thickening. A high RI (> 0.90) is also associated with acute rejection.

2.125 Chronic renal transplant rejection appears sonographically as:
    A. a decrease in cortical echoes
    B. a well-defined renal sinus
    C. a loss of distinction between cortex and medulla
    D. a decrease in renal size
    E. A and C
    F. C and D
    G. B and C

F is correct.
In chronic rejection, the kidney becomes small and has an irregular contour; there is a loss of distinction of internal renal architecture.

Lower urinary tract

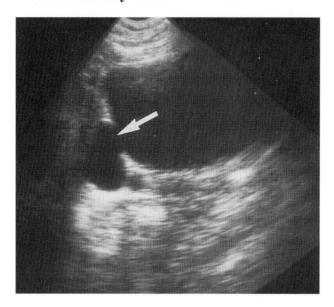

Use the above scan to answer question 2.126.

2.126 This pelvic sonogram was taken of an asymptomatic patient. (Please don't tell the HMO!) What is YOUR impression?
  A. ureterocele
  B. ovarian cyst
  C. bladder diverticulum
  D. urachal cyst

C is correct.
Bladder diverticula, or outpouchings of the bladder wall, may be congenital or due to acquired lesions. Filled with urine, they appear anechoic with good transonicity. Careful scanning demonstrates the connection between a diverticulum and the bladder. They usually empty when the patient voids but, if urinary stasis occurs, they may be a source of infection. A **ureterocele** is a cyst-like enlargement of the lower portion of the ureter that may obstruct the ureterovesicular junction. A **urachal cyst** is a congenital anomaly that arises when the allantoic canal fails to close in a fetus. It maintains its connection with the bladder and may become infected. It is located anterosuperior to the bladder, not lateral as in this case.

2.127 A urinary tract congenital anomaly specific to MEN only is:
  A. ureterocele
  B. diverticula
  C. posterior urethral valves
  D. urachal cysts
  E. bladder tumors

C is correct.
Posterior urethral valves, an obstruction in the prostatic urethra originating near the verumontanum, may result in dilatation of the urethra, bladder wall hypertrophy, hydroureter and hydronephrosis.

2.128 Ureteral jets:
  A. are caused by reflux of urine into the ureter
  B. only occur rarely
  C. are thought to be caused by urine sprayed in from the ureters into the static urine of the bladder
  D. are a pathologic condition
  E. take off from La Guardia Airport

C is correct.
Ureteral jets are seen every 5–20 s and last from a fraction of a second to up to 3 s. Each ureter functions independently of the other. The jet starts in the area of the ureteral orifice and flows toward the center of the bladder. Studies have shown that the ureteral jet flow is impaired in abnormalities that obstruct the ureter and by abnormal ureteral peristalsis.

2.129 The severity of a bladder tumor depends on:
  A. whether it has calcified
  B. its size alone
  C. whether it has metastasized
  D. how deeply it has invaded the bladder wall
  E. C and D
  F. A, B and C
  G. A and B

E is correct.
For curability, it has been found that the single most important factor is the depth that the tumor has invaded the bladder wall. Other factors include grade of malignancy and histologic type of the tumor.

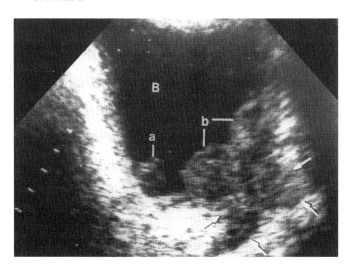

Use the above scan to answer question 2.130.

2.130 Mr O, a 55-year-old martini-mixer, presented with painless hematuria. What is the MOST likely diagnosis after this sonographic evaluation?
  A. squamous cell carcinoma
  B. bladderstones
  C. transitional cell carcinoma
  D. leiomyoma
  E. adenocarcinoma

C is correct.
Transitional cell carcinomas constitute 90% of bladder tumors. They often present with painless hematuria in the group ages 40–60 years, with a male predominance of 3:1. These lesions vary greatly in appearance, ranging from villous tufts to papillary growths with fronds to nodular infiltrating tumors.

2.131 Calculi in the urinary bladder:
  A. may be caused by a Foley catheter
  B. may be caused by a urea-splitting microorganism
  C. always pass into the bladder from the upper urinary tract
  D. display posterior enhancement
  E. A, B and C
  F. A and B
  G. A and D

F is correct.
An intravesicular foreign body, such as a Foley catheter, may become encrusted with calcium salts. Infection by *Proteus mirabilis* has also been shown to be linked to stone formation. Bladder calculi may form within the bladder itself or come from the kidneys. They demonstrate acoustic shadowing as do stones elsewhere in the body.

Normal retroperitoneum

2.132 The retroperitoneum:
  A. is lined with parietal peritoneum
  B. is covered anteriorly with parietal peritoneum
  C. is composed of the greater and lesser sacs
  D. is the potential space between the visceral and parietal peritoneum

B is correct.
The retroperitoneum lies posterior to the peritoneal cavity and, hence, is only covered in front by the peritoneal membrane. The greater and lesser sacs are compartments of the peritoneal cavity, which is the potential space between visceral and parietal peritoneum.

2.133 Which of the following organs are located retroperitoneally?
  A. pancreas, stomach and spleen
  B. pancreas, kidneys and spleen
  C. pancreas, kidneys and adrenal glands
  D. stomach, spleen and liver
  E. aorta, inferior vena cava and main portal vein

C is correct.
The stomach, spleen and liver are intraperitoneal organs. The main portal vein is intraperitoneal where it enters the porta hepatis.

2.134 The space of the retroperitoneum in which the adrenal glands are located is the:
  A. posterior pararenal space
  B. anterior pararenal space
  C. perirenal space
  D. space in which the IVC and aorta are found

C is correct.
The perirenal space contains the kidneys, adrenals and perinephric fat, and is bounded by Gerota's fascia. The anterior pararenal space contains the pancreas, duodenal sweep, and ascending and descending colons. The posterior pararenal space lies posterior to Gerota's fascia and anterior to the transversalis fascia, and contains the psoas and quadratus lumborum muscles. The IVC and aorta reside in the unnamed retroperitoneal spaces.

2.135 With the exception of the pancreas, patient preparation for a retroperitoneal sonogram includes:
  A. NPO for 6–8 hours
  B. administration of antacids
  C. no preparation
  D. 4–6 glasses of water
  E. an enema

C is correct.
Since these areas are posterior in the body, no patient preparation is necessary. The pancreas, although retroperitoneal, is fairly close to the anterior wall of the abdomen. As the body and tail of the pancreas are near the stomach, NPO and a water-filled stomach are often necessary for optimal visualization of this organ.

2.136 When scanning the right adrenal gland, it is helpful to:
- A. use the aorta as an anatomic landmark
- B. scan transversely posterior to the IVC
- C. locate the right diaphragmatic crus
- D. scan intercostally with the patient LLD
- E. A and D
- F. B, C and D
- G. A and C

F is correct.
The adrenal glands, which are small and homogeneously hypoechoic, are difficult to visualize sonographically. Only by using the anatomic landmarks and careful scanning can they be distinguished.

Retroperitoneal pathology

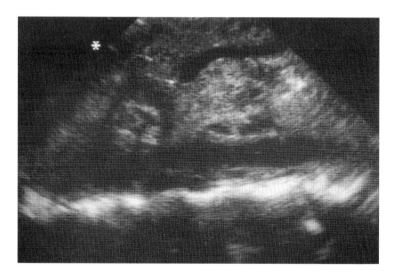

Use the above scan to answer question 2.137.

2.137 What evidence of retroperitoneal pathology is seen in this sonogram?
- A. anterior displacement of the IVC
- B. lateral displacement of the aorta
- C. anterior displacement of the SMA
- D. hydronephrosis

C is correct.
All of these are possibilities in retroperitoneal pathology. Hydronephrosis may be caused by tumors or enlarged lymph nodes compressing the ureters.

2.138 Pathology causing enlargement in the left adrenal gland may result in:
- A. a pressure deformity of the upper pole of the left kidney
- B. anterior displacement of the IVC
- C. medial displacement of the aorta
- D. right flank pain
- E. A and D
- F. A and C
- G. B and C

F is correct.
One of the greatest diagnostic challenges is differentiating an adrenal mass from a mass in the upper pole of a kidney. Patient history is most important, and should include the patient's symptoms, blood test results, blood pressure changes and findings with other imaging modalities.

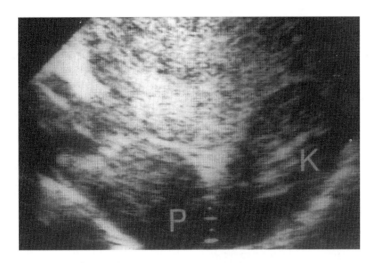

Use the above scan to answer question 2.139.

2.139 This is a sonogram of a 50-year-old patient who presented with a palpable lumbar mass and episodic hypertension. The MOST likely diagnosis is:
   A. nephroblastoma
   B. pheochromocytoma
   C. carcinoma
   D. lymphoma
   E. sarcoma

B is correct.
Pheochromocytomas usually originate from the chromaffin cells in the adrenal medulla. These tumors are generally large well-encapsulated solids; 90% are benign, and patient symptoms include chronic or episodic hypertension, headaches, sweating and elevated levels of urinary catecholamines.

2.140 A 6-month-old boy presented with a large abdominal mass. His sonogram revealed a complex echogenic tumor with poorly defined borders. Unfortunately, an MRI scan demonstrated extension of this tumor into the chest. The MOST likely diagnosis is:
   A. nephroblastoma
   B. hepatocellular carcinoma
   C. hypernephroma
   D. neuroblastoma

D is correct.
Neuroblastomas are tumors that occur in infancy, usually originating from the neural tissue of the adrenal glands. These tumors may also arise from the sympathetic ganglia in the neck, chest and abdomen. They are not as well circumscribed as Wilms' tumors, and may rapidly spread beyond the adrenal gland. Calcifications are also a common finding in neuroblastomas, but are much less common in Wilms' tumors. The peak incidence for Wilms' tumors is at ages 2–3 years.

2.141 An adrenal mass that causes hyperbilirubinemia in neonates after a difficult delivery is:
   A. Wilms' tumor
   B. pheochromocytoma
   C. hemorrhage
   D. nephroblastoma
   E. hydronephrosis

C is correct.
Neonatal adrenals are relatively large and have a highly engorged vascular cortex. Birth trauma, anoxia or systemic disorders, such as thrombocytopenia purpura, may cause hemorrhage; 70% occur on the right side and may result in biliary obstruction. The sonographic appearance of the hemorrhage ranges from cystic to complex, depending on the age of the bleed.

2.142 Mr. S presented with abdominal pain, diabetes mellitus, weakened muscles and elastic tissue in the body. His sonogram revealed a solid mass in his lumbar region. The MOST likely diagnosis is:
   A. adrenal pheochromocytoma
   B. adrenocortical carcinoma
   C. hypernephroma
   D. Wilms' tumor

B is correct.
Ninety percent of adrenocortical carcinomas produce steroids, causing symptoms similar to Cushing's disease. With increased cortisol production, there is an increase in gluconeogenesis by the liver. The islets of Langerhans cannot produce enough insulin, and diabetes mellitus results. Sonographically, adrenocortical carcinomas appear solid or complex, with zones of hemorrhage and necrosis. They tend to invade the adrenal veins, IVC and lymph nodes. Vascular invasion helps to distinguish them from benign adrenal tumors.

2.143 A primary retroperitoneal tumor that is found somewhat more frequently in men and presents primarily in the fifth to seventh decades is:
   A. rhabdomyosarcoma
   B. leiomyoma
   C. malignant histiosarcoma
   D. retroperitoneal seeding

C is correct.
Sarcomas are tumors derived from mesenchymal tissue. Histiosarcomas appear as well-defined masses with variable echo patterns. Rhabdomyosarcomas appear to be less well-defined, very invasive and spread into adjoining soft tissue. Retroperitoneal seeding occurs when other tumors metastasize and begin to grow on the retroperitoneal lining.

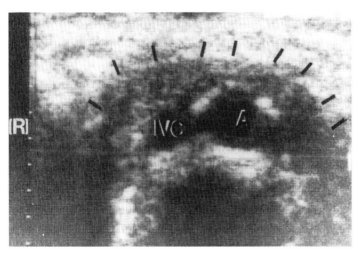

Use the above scan to answer question 2.144.

2.144 This sonogram is of Mr. C, a 55-year-old man who presented with back and flank pain, weight loss, nausea and vomiting, malaise, hypertension and anuria. The MOST likely diagnosis is:
   A. retroperitoneal seeding
   B. rhabdomyosarcoma
   C. adrenal carcinoma
   D. retroperitoneal fibrosis

D is correct.
Retroperitoneal fibrosis (dense fibrous tissue proliferation) appears sonographically as large bulky hypoechoic masses with ill-defined irregular margins. The etiology is either unknown, or is associated with patients who have known retroperitoneal malignancies or who are treated with the drug methysergide, which is used in the treatment of migraine.

2.145 The most common primary malignant, retroperitoneal, soft-tissue tumor in adults is:
    A. rhabdomyosarcoma
    B. liposarcoma
    C. leiomyosarcoma
    D. lipoma

B is correct.
Liposarcomas appear sonographically as very echogenic solid masses. As with the other retroperitoneal tumors listed, they may grow to an immense size before they are clinically detected. Leiomyosarcomas may arise retroperitoneally, but are more often found in the uterus and gastrointestinal tract. Lipomas are the benign form of liposarcomas.

2.146 Mr. G suffered a bout of pyelonephritis. Clinically, he presented with fever and an elevated white cell count. An ill-defined hypoechoic lesion with good transonicity was observed adjacent to the lower pole of his right kidney. The MOST likely diagnosis is:
    A. pancreatic pseudocyst
    B. urinoma
    C. lymphoma
    D. abscess

D is correct.
An abscess is a pus-filled inflammatory mass found most commonly in patients who have had surgical operations, recent perforation of the gastrointestinal tract, or inflammation of the kidneys or pancreas. They are usually hypoechoic but, occasionally, appear to be highly echogenic due to the presence of gas-producing microorganisms.

2.147 A patient diagnosed with AIDS should be screened sonographically for:
    A. lymphoma
    B. retroperitoneal abscess
    C. splenomegaly
    D. gallstones
    E. hydronephrosis
    F. A and C
    G. A, B and C
    H. B and E

F is correct.
AIDS, a disease characterized by destruction of the immune system, results in the development of many infectious and neoplastic processes, including cytomegalovirus and herpesvirus infections, cryptococcosis, candidiasis, Kaposi's sarcoma and lymphoma.

2.148 A multiseptate cystic-like mass in the peritoneal cavity that arises from mucinous tumors is:
    A. benign cystic teratoma
    B. pseudomyxoma peritonei
    C. abscess
    D. lymphocele
    E. urinoma

B is correct.
Pseudomyxoma peritonei arises from mucin-producing tumors of the ovary and appendix. The peritoneal cavity is filled with a gel-like substance that could be mistaken for ascites.

Spleen

2.149 Which of the following is MOST likely to result in an enlarged spleen?
    A. portal hypertension
    B. renal vein thrombosis
    C. severe sickle cell anemia
    D. hepatopetal blood flow

A is correct.
Portal hypertension is usually the result of liver disease (e.g. cirrhosis) which impedes the flow of blood in the liver. In very severe portal hypertension, the blood flow becomes hepato-fugal – blood flows away from the liver. This reversal of flow in the splenic vein causes splenomegaly. (Hepatopetal means flow of blood towards the liver.) In severe sickle cell disease, the spleen eventually shrinks to become smaller than normal and is non-functional because of repeated infarctions.

2.150 A normal spleen demonstrates an echogenicity equal to or slightly less than that of the:
   A. pancreas
   B. renal cortex
   C. renal medulla
   D. liver

D is correct.
The spleen is usually more echogenic than either the renal medulla or cortex and less echogenic than the pancreas.

2.151 Of the following, the OPTIMAL technique for scanning the spleen is:
   A. intercostally through ribs 7 and 8
   B. intercostally through ribs 10 and 11
   C. intercostally with the patient in the LLD position
   D. subcostally with the patient supine

B is correct.
The spleen lies in the left hypochondriac region along the axis of the tenth vertebra. Usually, the best way to scan is intercostally, with the patient RLD and NPO. This minimizes bowel gas from the stomach.

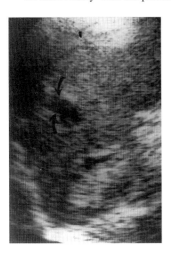

Use the above scan to answer question 2.152.

2.152 Joe Wyoming received a hard blow in the left hypochondrium. Sophie the sonographer came to his rescue. This is the sonogram taken by Sophie of his spleen. What is the MOST likely diagnosis?
   A. splenic infarction
   B. histoplasmosis
   C. splenic hematoma
   D. normal spleen

C is correct.
The spleen is an organ that may be injured as a result of blunt trauma. A fresh hematoma may not show up sonographically as it may be isoechoic to the splenic parenchyma. The hematoma changes from isoechoic to cystic to more echogenic as the hematoma organizes and undergoes clotting. A hematoma may be located within the spleen, as shown here, or may be found between the spleen and its capsule – 'subcapsular'. When it is subcapsular, it may have a crescentic shape.

2.153 When the spleen is located in an ectopic position due to extreme weight loss or prune-belly syndrome, this is termed:
   A. an accessory spleen
   B. a born-again spleen
   C. a wandering spleen
   D. an aplastic spleen

C is correct.
A wandering spleen in an ectopic position is due to stretching of the supportive ligaments of the spleen. Accessory spleens are extra spleens, usually located in the splenic hilus.
A born-again spleen occurs following a splenectomy, when small accessory spleens enlarge to assume normal splenic functions.

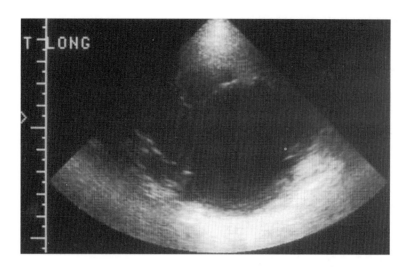

Use the above scan to answer question 2.154.

2.154 This is a sonogram of the spleen taken in an asymptomatic patient. What is the MOST likely diagnosis?
    A. focal abscess
    B. congenital cyst
    C. epidermoid cyst
    D. echinococcal cyst

D is correct.
Parasitic cysts are the most common benign cysts worldwide. They are usually of *Echinococcus* (hydatid) origin. Sonographically, they may vary from simple cysts to those with infolding membranes and hydatid sand (debris). They usually demonstrate a well-defined posterior wall and posterior enhancement. These cysts may be seen concurrently in the liver. Congenital splenic cysts are rare. Epidermoid or epithelial cysts constitute around 10% of non-parasitic cysts. They develop mainly before 20 years of age, and originate from the splenic capsular mesothelium, which undergoes cystic dilation and occasional metaplasia.

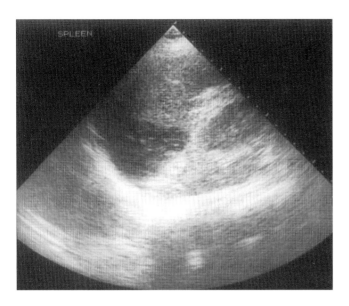

SPLEEN

Use the above scan to answer question 2.155.

2.155 A patient presented with sudden left upper quadrant pain. This sonogram visualizes a well-demarcated wedge-shaped region in the periphery of the spleen. The MOST likely diagnosis is:
  A. focal abscess
  B. infarction
  C. rupture
  D. lymphoma

B is correct.
Splenic infarctions are the sequelae to many different pathologic etiologies, including bacterial endocarditis, tumor embolization and leukemia. They present with sudden pain and have been described as having two phases: an acute inflammatory phase, where they appear to be hypoechoic and homogeneous; and a necrotic phase, where they appear to be more echogenic and heterogeneous. A splenic rupture usually occurs after blunt abdominal trauma. A sonographer should look for an enlarging and heterogeneous spleen with possible subcapsular hematomas. If the spleen is ruptured, free blood may also be present in the flanks, Morrison's pouch and in the pelvis.

2.156 In a patient with AIDS, the spleen often appears:
  A. enlarged
  B. shrunken
  C. with multiple hemangiomas
  D. with numerous punctate non-shadowing echogenic foci
  E. A and C
  F. A and D
  G. C and D

F is correct.
AIDS often occurs with extrapulmonary *Pneumocystis carinii* deposition, which presents as tiny calcific granulomata scattered throughout the spleen, liver, kidneys, adrenals and pancreas. These tiny non-shadowing calcifications may also be found as a remnant of histoplasmosis or tuberculosis infection. Fungal infections such as candidiasis may also be found in AIDS and other immunosuppressed patients. Hemangiomas are hyperechoic vascular tumors that are usually benign.

2.157 Mr. M was found to have a markedly enlarged liver and spleen on his sonogram of the upper abdomen. Focal hypoechoic and hyperechoic areas with no acoustic shadowing were visualized throughout the spleen and liver. The MOST likely diagnosis is:
   A. AIDS
   B. Gaucher's disease
   C. metastases from the gastrointestinal tract
   D. multiple abscesses

B is correct.
Gaucher's disease is a genetic disorder in which an enzyme deficiency causes accumulation of glucocerebrosides in the reticuloendothelial cells.

2.158 Repeated splenic infarctions may result in:
   A. a small fibrotic spleen as seen in sickle cell disease
   B. an enlarged spleen as seen in sickle cell disease
   C. an enlarged spleen as seen in splenic metastases
   D. an enlarged spleen as seen in Hodgkin's disease

A is correct.
In sickle cell anemia, repeated infarctions result in non-functional, small, fibrotic spleens. Calcifications are also often present. Splenic metastases and Hodgkin's disease are associated with enlargement, but not as a result of an infarction process.

2.159 When multiple tumor-like nodules occur in the spleen, the MOST likely diagnosis is:
   A. a primary angiosarcoma
   B. lymphomatous metastases
   C. primary hemangioma
   D. *Histoplasmosis* infection

B is correct.
Hodgkin's lymphoma usually begins in the lymph nodes and then spreads to the spleen. Sonographically, lesions may appear to be either hypo- or hyperechoic nodules and may or may not cause diffuse enlargement. Angiosarcoma is a rare malignant primary tumor in the spleen. It affects men and women equally, and presents sonographically as large nodular, heterogeneous, solid masses in the left upper quadrant.

Abdominal aorta

2.160 With regard to the abdominal aorta, which of the following is FALSE?
   A. it has a thicker tunica media than the IVC
   B. as it courses inferiorly, it becomes more anterior in the body
   C. the first major vessel that it gives rise to in the abdomen is the celiac axis
   D. as it courses inferiorly, it becomes more posterior in the body

D is correct.
The abdominal aorta courses from a posterior position at the diaphragm to a more anterior position at the umbilicus. It follows the curvature of the spine.

2.161 Which of the following is TRUE for branching of the aorta from superior to inferior?
   A. superior mesenteric artery, inferior mesenteric artery, renal arteries
   B. superior mesenteric artery, celiac artery, common iliac artery
   C. celiac artery, superior mesenteric artery, inferior mesenteric artery
   D. inferior phrenic artery, renal artery, celiac artery

C is correct.
These are the three largest anterior visceral arteries arising from the abdominal aorta. The renal arteries arise laterally from the aorta at approximately the level of the superior mesenteric artery.

2.162 A color Doppler scan of a normal abdominal aorta demonstrates:
   A. plug flow
   B. parabolic flow
   C. stenotic flow
   D. turbulent flow

A is correct.
In plug flow, the column of blood travels at nearly the same velocity at the center of a large vessel as it does peripherally near the wall. Parabolic flow, with the greatest velocity in the center and the lowest flow along the walls, is seen in smaller vessels. Stenotic flow occurs when there is narrowing of a vessel.

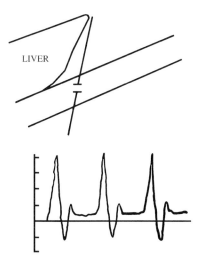

Use the above diagram to answer question 2.163.

2.163 This duplex Doppler scan of the abdominal aorta demonstrates:
   A. diphasic low-resistance flow
   B. triphasic high-resistance flow
   C. diphasic high-resistance flow
   D. low impedance waveform with prominent diastolic flow

B is correct.
Because of the large amount of elastic connective tissue in the aorta, the vessel has a high resistance or impedance. The three phases of flow are: systole; a small reverse flow; and diastole. Choice D is characteristic of the renal arteries.

2.164 To measure a true transverse diameter of a tortuous aorta, the BEST method is to:
   A. position the patient in RLD
   B. rotate the transducer 90° from the parasagittal plane of the aorta
   C. rotate the transducer 180° from the parasagittal plane of the aorta
   D. position the transducer in a true transverse plane to the upper abdomen

B is correct.
As the aorta is tortuous (twisty and turning), a true transverse of the abdomen will not yield a true transverse of the vessel.

2.165 On color Doppler, a tortuous aorta presents as:
   A. red and blue disorganized flow
   B. only blue flow
   C. only red flow
   D. no flow

A is correct.
Tortuosity leads to turbulent flow represented by a mixing of color.

2.166 The anteroposterior caliber of a normal aorta just before the bifurcation is:
- A. 2.4 cm
- B. 1.5 mm
- C. 1.5 cm
- D. 1.8 cm

C is correct.

A normal abdominal aorta measures approximately 2.4 cm at rib 11, 2.1 cm above the renal arteries, 1.8 cm below the renal arteries and 1.5 cm just above the bifurcation.

2.167 In the majority of the population, the celiac axis:
- A. bifurcates into the splenic and common hepatic arteries
- B. bifurcates into the left gastric and proper hepatic arteries
- C. trifurcates into the splenic, common hepatic and left gastric arteries
- D. trifurcates into the splenic, common hepatic and right gastric arteries

C is correct.

The branching scheme of the celiac axis is: 1) splenic artery; 2) common hepatic artery > proper hepatic artery > left and right hepatic arteries > right gastric artery > gastroduodenal artery; and 3) left gastric artery.

2.168 The most common cause of abdominal aortic aneurysm is:
- A. cystic medial necrosis
- B. syphilis
- C. atherosclerosis
- D. of unknown etiology

C is correct.

An aneurysm is an abnormal localized dilatation of an artery. Aortic aneurysms are found in a male-to-female ratio of 5:1, especially in the group aged > 50 years old. Atherosclerosis is responsible for approximately 90% of abdominal aortic aneurysms. Syphilis is associated with some aneurysms of the thoracic aorta. Cystic medial necrosis may also be an underlying cause.

2.169 The most common presenting symptom in abdominal aortic aneurysm rupture is:
- A. right upper quadrant pain
- B. pulsatile mass on physical examination
- C. acute abdominal pain
- D. no symptoms

C is correct.

A ruptured aneurysm usually presents with acute abdominal pain and shock, and may present with an expanding abdominal mass. In contrast, an unruptured aneurysm is most often asymptomatic; however, most of these are palpable as pulsatile masses.

2.170 In aortic ectasia, there is:
- A. widening of normal aortic diameter up to 3.0 cm
- B. widening of normal aortic diameter up to 2.5 cm
- C. narrowing of the aortic diameter
- D. aneurysmal dilatation of the aorta to > 3.5 cm

A is correct.

Ectasia is defined as a slight widening of the aorta up to 3.0 cm. Aortic wall irregularities due to calcific changes may also be detected.

2.171 Aortic thrombi:
- A. always result when there is aneurysm formation
- B. usually form on the anterior and lateral walls of an aneurysm
- C. cause the true lumen of the vessel to become narrowed
- D. usually form on the posterior wall of an aneurysm
- E. cause the true lumen of the vessel to be widened
- F. C and D
- G. B and C

G is correct.

Thrombi typically produce low-level echoes and occasionally contain calcifications. Reverberations from a calcific anterior vessel wall may obscure a thrombus. If a thrombus is suspected and not detected on 2-D sonography, Doppler interrogation of the region is confirmatory if there is absence of flow in the region of the thrombus. A clot causes narrowing of the true lumen, and typical stenotic flow with increased velocity can be measured.

THE ABDOMEN (AND SMALL PARTS) 91

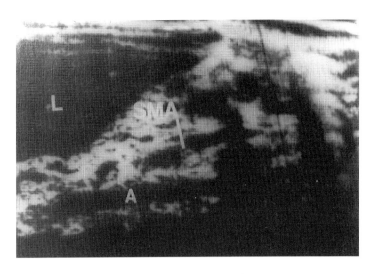

Use the above scan to answer question 2.172.

2.172 This sonogram of the upper abdomen displays:
   A. an aortic dissection
   B. an aortic aneurysm with a clot-filled lumen
   C. a narrowed aorta
   D. a saccular aneurysm

C is correct.
Takayasu's arteritis causes narrowing throughout the length of the aorta.

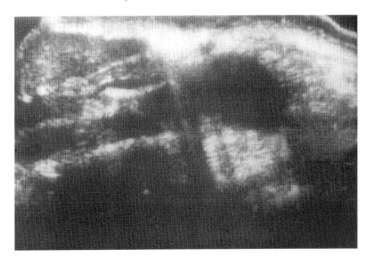

Use the above scan to answer question 2.173.

2.173 This sonogram depicts a(n):
   A. saccular aneurysm
   B. fusiform aneurysm
   C. dissecting aneurysm
   D. ectatic aorta

B is correct.
Fusiform aneurysms are the most common type of abdominal aortic aneurysm. They may present as spindles, which may be eccentric to one side, or as cylinders, when expansion of the vessel is uniform. Fusiform aneurysms may be as long as 20 cm and may extend into the renal and common iliac arteries.

2.174 A saccular aneurysm may be difficult to detect because:
    A. its connection to the aorta may not be easily visualized
    B. it may be confused with a pseudoaneurysm
    C. it may be confused with a dissecting aneurysm
    D. it may be confused with lymphadenopathy
    E. A, B and D
    F. A, B and C

E is correct.
All of these are pitfalls in trying to detect saccular aneurysms. Interrogation with color may resolve some of these possible differential diagnoses.

2.175 In the range of 3.5–5.9 cm, the average yearly growth of an aortic aneurysm is:
    A. 3.0 cm
    B. 0.23–0.28 cm
    C. 3.5–4.0 cm
    D. 4.5–5.0 cm

B is correct.
Research has shown that this is the normal rate of growth. It is recommended that patients be clinically monitored by ultrasound examination; if the growth rate is higher than this, more aggressive treatment may be indicated.

2.176 The MOST common location for an aortic dissection is:
    A. in the abdominal aorta above the renal arteries
    B. in the ascending thoracic aorta
    C. in the descending thoracic aorta
    D. in the abdominal aorta below the renal arteries

B is correct.
Aortic dissections, caused by hypertension, cystic medial necrosis or Marfan's syndrome, among others, are mainly found in the ascending thoracic aorta, but may extend down to the abdominal aorta. The most affected population is male (at a ratio of 2–3:1) ages 40–60 years and those with hypertension.

Gastrointestinal tract

2.177 Using an endoluminal transducer, the innermost layer of bowel wall is _____ and appears sonographically as _____.
    A. lamina propria, a hypoechoic layer
    B. mucosa-fluid interface, an echogenic line
    C. submucosa, an echogenic layer
    D. serosa, an echogenic layer

B is correct.
With an endoluminal transducer, the layers of bowel seen, from inner to outer, are:
1) mucosa–fluid interface: echogenic line;
2) deeper mucosa, lamina propria, muscularis mucosa: hypoechoic layer; 3) submucosa: echogenic layer; 4) muscularis propria: hypoechoic layer; and 5) serosa: thin echogenic layer

2.178 The simplest means for a sonographer to ascertain whether a cystic-like structure in the left upper quadrant is the stomach is to:
    A. administer a few sips of water through a straw, then turn the patient LLD
    B. have the patient in the supine position
    C. look for peristalsis
    D. administer a few sips of water through a straw, then turn the patient RLD

D is correct.
The water produces a bubbly pattern in the stomach. When the patient is turned RLD, the gas in the antrum of the stomach is replaced by water, thus providing good visualization and identification.

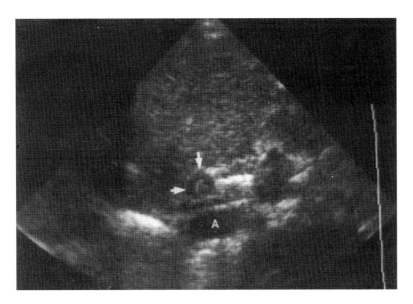

Use the above scan to answer question 2.179.

2.179 The portion(s) of the gastrointestinal tract shown in this sonogram is / are _____ described as _____.

    A. a telescoped bowel, the pseudokidney sign
    B. the gastroesophageal junction, the target sign
    C. the small bowel, the keyboard sign
    D. the stomach and esophagus, the double-bubble sign

B is correct.
The mucus within the lumen gives an echogenic appearance. This is surrounded by the bowel wall, which appears as a hypoechoic rim. An intussuscepted, telescoped bowel may appear either as a large target sign or a pseudokidney sign, depending on the plane of visualization. The keyboard sign represents the valvulae conniventes of the small bowel. The double-bubble sign is seen either *in utero* or in neonates when there is duodenal atresia. Fluid is backed-up in the proximal duodenum and stomach, thus creating a 'double bubble'.

2.180 The most common primary malignant tumor in the stomach is:
    A. colonic carcinoma
    B. gastric leiomyoma
    C. gastric carcinoma
    D. gastric adenoma

C is correct.
Gastric carcinoma is the third most common gastrointestinal malignancy following colonic cancer and pancreatic carcinoma. It arises from the gastric mucosa, and invades the submucosa and muscularis layers. Tumors range from focal polypoid masses to invasion of the entire stomach.

2.181 Appendicitis may be diagnosed with 80–90% accuracy with sonography when:
    A. the appendix measures > 6 mm in diameter
    B. the appendix measures > 6 cm in diameter
    C. the appendix measures 8–10 cm in length
    D. the appendix is located retrocecally

A is correct.
Other sonographic findings in acute appendicitis may include wall thickness > 3 mm and the presence of an appendicolith. A normal appendix measures 8–10 cm in length, although this varies. When the appendix is located behind the cecum (retrocecal), it is difficult to visualize sonographically.

2.182 Acute appendicitis may present with which of the following manifestations?

    A right upper quadrant pain

    B. leukocytosis

    C. nausea

    D. periumbilical pain

    E. A and D

    F. all of the above

F is correct.

2.183 A perforated appendix:

    A. appears highly edematous sonographically

    B. always demonstrates calcified appendicoliths

    C. may appear normal sonographically

    D. has a distended lumen

C is correct.

Once rupture has occurred, the lumen is no longer distended and the diagnosis is difficult to make with ultrasound. The presence of calcified appendicoliths strongly suggests appendicitis, but they are **not always** present. (On perforation, a localized walled-off abscess results.) Rarely, on rupture of an appendix that is filled with mucus, a gelatinous ascites called pseudomyxomatous peritonei fills the abdominopelvic cavity.

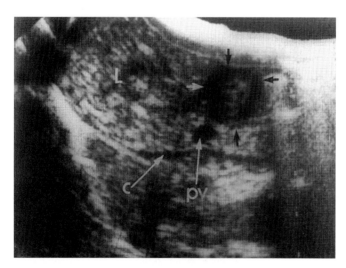

Use the above scan to answer question 2.184.

2.184 Baby Hughie is 1 week old and already giving his parents a hard time. He takes very little when feeding, then vomits vigorously, soiling everything within 10 feet of him. Frantic, his parents take him for an upper abdominal sonogram. This sonogram clearly demonstrates:

    A. a stomach ulcer

    B. duodenal atresia

    C. intussusception

    D. hypertrophic pyloric stenosis

D is correct.

Hypertrophic pyloric stenosis (HPS) is familial, and found in a male-to-female ratio of 4:1. Discovered within the first few weeks of life, symptoms and signs include non-bilious projectile vomiting, dehydration, poor weight gain and palpation of an olive-shaped mass in the abdomen. The parameters pathognomonic for HPS are: wall thickness > 4 mm; pyloric diameter > 15 mm; and pyloric length > 20 mm. The stomach is often filled with liquid due to obstruction of the pylorus portion.

2.185 A sonogram of the ileum of a patient with non-specific pelvic pain reveals a hypoechoic thickening of the bowel wall and mesentery. The MOST likely (but not only) diagnosis is:
   A. a bowel tumor
   B. appendicitis
   C. Crohn's disease
   D. pericecal abscess

C is correct.
Crohn's disease is a granulomatous inflammatory disease affecting the terminal ileum and colon. The bowel may form fibrosing strictures and fistulas to other parts of the bowel, urinary bladder or perineum. Ultrasound characteristics are symmetrical thickening of the bowel wall, especially the mucosal and submucosal layers.

2.186 In the condition of ileus:
   A. the colon becomes distended with fluid
   B. the bowel becomes distended with either air or fluid
   C. there is acute intestinal obstruction
   D. the small bowel is floating in ascites

B is correct.
Ileus is a pseudo-obstruction of the bowel due to decreased motility. The etiology is varied, including peritonitis, spinal fracture, renal colic, bowel ischemia and infection. It is normally seen postsurgically.

2.187 In a patient who has superior mesenteric artery (SMA) syndrome, sonographic findings may:
   A. disappear when the patient is in a prone position
   B. include a dilated, fluid-filled second portion of duodenum
   C. include an aneurysmal SMA
   D. include a dilated third portion of duodenum
   E. A and C
   F. A and B

F is correct.
In this syndrome, the stomach and duodenum may be dilated proximal to the point where the superior mesenteric vessels indent the duodenum. These findings are seen when the patient is supine and disappear when the patient is prone because, in this position, the SMA no longer presses on the gastrointestinal tract. This syndrome is more common in very thin patients, and in those who have extensive burns or acute pancreatitis.

Thyroid and parathyroid glands

2.188 When scanning the thyroid gland, the common carotid artery and jugular vein are seen:
   A. anterolaterally
   B. anteromedially
   C. posteromedially
   D. posterolaterally

D is correct.
These vessels are located in the carotid sheath along with the vagus nerve. They are easily visualized by their anechoic interiors and echogenic walls.

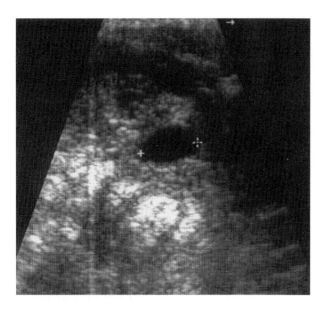

Use the above scan to answer question 2.189.

2.189 In this sonogram:
  A. a cystic mass is seen on the anterior aspect of the right lateral lobe of the thyroid
  B. a cystic mass is seen on the posterior aspect of the right lateral lobe of the thyroid
  C. an isoechoic mass is seen on the anterior aspect of the right lateral lobe of the thyroid
  D. a cystic mass is seen on the posterior aspect of the left lateral lobe of the thyroid

B is correct.
The mass is well-circumscribed and demonstrates good posterior enhancement. This meets the criteria for a thyroid cyst, but was diagnosed sonographically as cystic degeneration of an adenoma as other small nodules were identified in the left lateral lobe.

2.190 Mr. Miles has been ill for several months. His symptoms include fever and neck pain radiating to the jaw and ear. Sonographically, his thyroid appears to be diffusely enlarged and hypoechoic. The MOST likely diagnosis is:
  A. thyroid carcinoma
  B. acute thyroiditis
  C. subacute thyroiditis
  D. Hashimoto's thyroiditis

B is correct.
Acute thyroiditis is usually accompanied by fever and painful enlargement of the thyroid gland. Subacute thyroiditis, more commonly known as de Quervain's thyroiditis, presents with similar symptoms, but is usually self-limiting, lasting only several weeks. Hashimoto's (chronic) thyroiditis is an autoimmune progressive disease found mainly in women which often results in hypothyroidism. Physical symptoms are intolerance to cold, weakness, eyelid and facial droop, and dry skin.

2.191 The MOST common malignant tumor of the thyroid gland is:
- A. papillary carcinoma
- B. follicular carcinoma
- C. medullary carcinoma
- D. lymphoma

A is correct.

Papillary carcinoma is the most common malignant tumor of the thyroid gland, comprising 50–70% of all thyroid cancers. It is most common in young women in their childbearing years. Follicular carcinoma is more malignant than papillary and is found in the same population. Medullary carcinoma accounts for around 10% of cancers in the thyroid, and often appears in genetic syndromes along with other tumors of the endocrine glands. Lymphoma is a very uncommon thyroid cancer.

2.192 A cystic mass in the neck seen anterior and superior to the thyroid is MOST likely a:
- A. cystic hygroma
- B. thyroglossal duct cyst
- C. branchial cleft cyst
- D. thyroid cyst

B is correct.

A thyroglossal duct cyst is a remnant of the thyroglossal duct, which extends from the base of the tongue to the isthmus of the thyroid in the midline. Normally, it atrophies and is absent in adults. Sonographically, it may appear cystic or display echoes within if there is hemorrhage or colloidal debris. Branchial cleft cysts, also remnants of fetal development, lie directly below the angle of the mandible and anterior to the sternocleidomastoid muscle. These cysts generally appear cystic, but solid components may be seen if there is infection or hemorrhage. Cystic hygromas, or benign congenital masses often found in conjunction with Turner's syndrome, may occur anywhere, but are found most often in the posterior portion of the neck.

2.193 Parathyroid glands:
- A. are always located behind the thyroid gland
- B. are easily discernible from thyroid tissue
- C. when pathologic, often appear homogeneously hypoechoic compared with thyroid tissue
- D. when pathologic, present with hypervascularity on color Doppler sonography
- E. A and C
- F. A and D
- G. C and D

G is correct.

Normal parathyroid glands cannot be demonstrated even with high-frequency probes. They are usually located posterior to the thyroid, but may also be ectopically located anterior to the thyroid, or retrosternal or posterior to the pharynx, trachea or esophagus. Adenomas, hyperplasias and carcinomas have similar patterns of morphology and echogenicity.

Breast

2.194 In breast sonography, glandular tissue appears as:
   A. echogenic lines
   B. hypoechoic lobules
   C. echogenic tissue
   D. peripheral ducts

C is correct.

The sonographic pattern of breast parenchyma varies with age and the subject, and depends on the amount and distribution of fibrous, fatty and glandular tissues. Fibrous tissue is the most echogenic, followed by glandular, whereas fatty tissue gives a hypoechoic appearance. The ducts appear as tubular anechoic structures radiating from the nipple into the breast parenchyma.

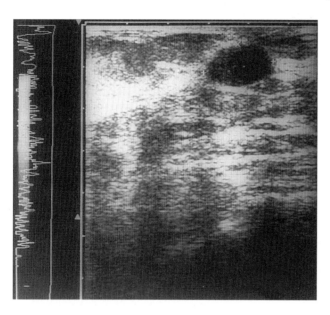

Use the above scan to answer question 2.195.

2.195 This sonogram of a breast mass meets the criteria for:
   A. a fibroadenoma
   B. an adenocarcinoma
   C. a cyst
   D. ductal ectasia

A is correct.

Fibroadenomas usually appear as well-circumscribed hypoechoic solid masses with poor through transmission. They may undergo necrosis and hyalinization, resulting in coarse 'popcorn' calcification.

Scrotum

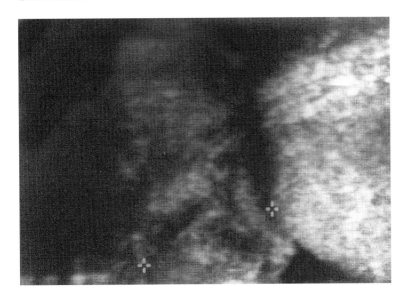

Use the above scan to answer question 2.196.

2.196 This scrotal sonogram MOST likely depicts:
    A. testicular torsion
    B. acute epididymitis
    C. testicular trauma
    D. malignant germ cell tumor

B is correct.
Epididymitis and/or orchitis are the most common infections involving the scrotum and the most common causes of acute scrotal pain. In most cases, the epididymis is enlarged and hypoechoic, and an accompanying hydrocele may be noted. Testicular torsion is best diagnosed sonographically by color Doppler, which can document incomplete or complete torsion (obstruction of blood to the testicle). Trauma to the testis may result in a hematocele, which may appear as a complex debris-filled fluid collection around the testis. Most scrotal tumors present as painless solid testicular masses with variable acoustic patterns.

2.197 Indication(s) for performing a scrotal sonogram for infertility include(s):
    A. acute scrotal pain
    B. palpable scrotal mass
    C. search for varicoceles
    D. search for undescended testis
    E. trauma
    F. A, C and E
    G. B and C
    H. C and D

H is correct.
There is a high risk of infertility with undescended testes that are not repaired before 6 years of age. Varicoceles in the scrotum increase the temperature and hamper spermatogenesis.

2.198 Testicular torsion may present with:
   A. acute pain with a complex debris-filled fluid
      collection around a testis
   B. a painless solid palpable mass in the testis
   C. an incomplete or complete cut-off of blood supply to
      the testicle
   D. a hydrocele around the testicle
   E. A, B and C
   F. C and D

F is correct.
Testicular torsion is best diagnosed sonographically by color Doppler, which can document
incomplete or complete torsion (interruption of
blood flow to the testicle). There may be an
associated hydrocele and scrotal skin thickening.
Trauma to the testis may result in a hematocele,
which may appear as a complex debris-filled
fluid collection around the testis. Most scrotal
tumors present as painless solid testicular masses
with variable acoustic patterns.

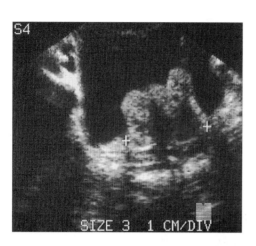

Use the above scan to answer question 2.199.

2.199 A 65-year-old man presented with frequent urination.
A sonogram of his kidneys revealed bilateral mild
hydronephrosis. Based on this pelvic sonogram, what
is the MOST likely diagnosis?
   A. bladder calculus
   B. benign prostatic hypertrophy
   C. prostatic cancer
   D. cystitis

B is correct.
Benign prostatic hypertrophy is the most
common cause of prostate enlargement in older
men. It may cause urethral obstruction, thereby
preventing complete emptying of the bladder.
Hydronephrosis may be a sequela of this
condition. Bladder cancer may also cause
hydronephrosis if the passage of urine is blocked
at the ureterovesical junction or urethral orifice.
Cystitis is inflammation of the bladder wall with
wall thickening.

2.200 Regarding primary testicular neoplasms, which of the
following statements is FALSE?
   A. Primary testicular cancer is the most common
      malignancy in men ages 20–35 years
   B. The most common sign of primary testicular cancer is
      painless enlargement of the testicle
   C. The most common ultrasound appearance of a
      seminoma is an ill-defined hyperechoic heterogeneous
      mass
   D. Undescended testes (cryptorchidism) are associated
      with a higher incidence of primary malignancies than
      are descended testes

C is correct.
The peak incidence of seminomas, the most
common primary malignancy of the testes, is in
young men. Sonographically, they appear as
hypoechoic homogeneous well-defined masses.

SECTION 3: OBSTETRICS AND GYNECOLOGY

More than one answer per question may be correct.

OBSTETRICS

First trimester

3.001 In an early gestation, the gestational sac:
A. represents the fluid-filled amniotic cavity
B. surrounds the decidua capsularis and decidua parietalis
C. can be visualized transvaginally by around 4 weeks and transabdominally by around 6 weeks
D. can be correlated with human chorionic gonadotropin (hCG) in the range of 300–750 milliunits/ml (I.U.; Second I.S.)

C and D are correct.
The early gestational sac represents the fluid-filled chorion, which contains the amniotic cavity, embryonic disc and yolk sac, and is surrounded by the decidua. A normal intra-uterine pregnancy should be visible using a transvaginal transducer at the serum hCG level given in choice D.

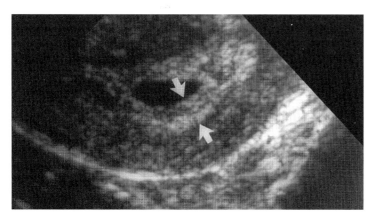

Use the above figure to answer question 3.002.

3.002 In this image, the arrows are pointing to a(n):
A. implantation bleed
B. single decidual sac
C. double decidual sac
D. early placenta

C is correct.
The placenta develops from the portion of the trophoblast attached to the myometrium, the decidua basalis. The double-sac sign represents two layers of gestational sac (decidua capsularis and decidua parietalis) before fusion. The decidua capsularis surrounds the developing gestational sac, and its presence suggests an intrauterine gestation. The amnion and chorion (within the gestational sac) fuse much later (at ± 16 weeks). Prior to fusion, the amniotic membrane may be seen separately within the gestational sac. An implantation bleed appears as a triangular hypoechoic or anechoic area outside of the gestational sac.

3.003 The echogenic secondary yolk sac is:
   A. the first structure to be seen within the gestational sac
   B. not visualized in an ectopic gestation
   C seen transabdominally at ± 4 weeks after the last menstrual period (LMP)
   D. is usually between 3–4 mm in diameter

A and D are correct.
The secondary yolk sac may be seen in ectopic pregnancies. Visualization of this echogenic circular structure may help to confirm either an intrauterine or an ectopic pregnancy, depending on its location The yolk sac is seen from ± 5 weeks transvaginally (6–7 weeks trans-abdominally) to ± 11 weeks.

3.004 An embryo (fetal pole) should be regularly imaged when the:
   A. gestational sac is 2.0 cm transvaginally
   B. yolk sac has not yet developed
   C. gestational sac is 2.5 cm transabdominally
   D. gestational sac is 2.0 cm transabdominally

A and C are correct.
The yolk sac is often the first structure seen in the gestational sac. With transabdominal scanning, a yolk sac can be visualized in a gestational sac > 2.0 cm, and a fetal pole can be seen in a gestational sac > 2.5 cm. If these structures cannot be seen at these times, it may be an indication of a blighted ovum.

3.005 During the first trimester, the developing embryo grows approximately _____ every day.
   A. 1–2 mm
   B. 2–3 mm
   C. 3–4 mm
   D. 4–5 mm

A is correct.
Differentiation between the head and body of the embryo can be made by 7–8 weeks; the ratio of head length-to-body length at that time is 1:2. Heart pulsations can usually be distinguished after 6 weeks.

3.006 On transvaginal imaging, by the end of the first trimester (11–13 weeks), the choroid plexus:
   A. is not present and cannot be imaged
   B. can be imaged as a hyperechoic structure in the lateral ventricle
   C. can be imaged as a hypoechoic structure in the lateral ventricle
   D. is seen as a linear echogenic structure in the gestational sac

B is correct.
Prior to week 10, the falx and choroid plexus are usually not present. If these structures are visible, the fetus is then at least 9 weeks old. At this time, the four-chambered heart may also be visualized, and the bones of the hands and feet imaged and evaluated.

3.007 A corpus luteum of pregnancy:
   A. is a functional cyst of the ovary
   B. precedes the formation of a follicular cyst
   C. becomes a corpus luteum cyst only if fertilization does not take place
   D. is 1.5–2.5 cm

A and D are correct.
On rupture of the dominant follicle in an ovary, the corpus luteum of menstruation may develop. It may appear echo-filled with thick borders. If it fails to involute (usually within 14 days), a 5–11-cm corpus luteum cyst may develop. If fertilization takes place, a corpus luteum cyst of pregnancy may develop, but generally resolves by 16 weeks. Hemorrhageor rupture may occur in these cysts.

3.008 A corpus luteum cyst of pregnancy is MOST likely to be seen:
   A. at 4–8 weeks
   B. at 8–16 weeks
   C. at 16–20 weeks
   D. throughout pregnancy

B is correct.
Normal-sized ovaries may be visualized during the first part of the first trimester. Corpus luteum cysts of pregnancy are generally unilocular and unilateral. There may below-level echoes within the cyst.

3.009 The posterior cul-de-sac contains a small amount of clear fluid, as seen on sonography. This is MOST likely to be evidence of:

    A. a normal situation

    B. an ectopic pregnancy

    C. pelvic inflammatory disease (PID)

    D. vesicouterine reflux

A is correct.

A small amount of clear fluid is sometimes visualized in the cul-de-sac (also called the pouch of Douglas or rectouterine pouch). With an ectopic pregnancy or PID, there is more likely be a larger, more complex, collection of fluid. Reflux does not appear in the cul-de-sac. The cul-de-sac is the most dependent part of the peritoneal cavity and may collect fluid due to any intra-abdominal cause. Fluid in this space must always be evaluated in light of the clinical situation.

3.010 A patient with a positive serum hCG test presents with some bleeding. The LMP indicates a 5–6-week gestation. Sonography indicates an empty gestational sac. The MOST likely diagnosis is a(n):

    A. blighted ovum

    B. complete spontaneous abortion

    C. ectopic pregnancy

    D. normal intrauterine gestation, but too early to detect the fetal pole

A and D are correct.

This most likely represents an intrauterine gestation when it is too early to see the fetus; a rescan is indicated. However, a blighted ovum cannot be ruled out on transabdominal examination unless the gestational sac is > 2.0 cm without a yolk sac or > 2.5 cm without a visualized embryonic heartbeat. An ectopic pregnancy may also be considered if a double decidual sac sign is not seen. In this case, evaluation of the adnexa and cul-de-sac is important. Complete spontaneous abortion is usually accompanied by profuse bleeding. Congenital heart disease is thought to be a factor in many spontaneous abortions.

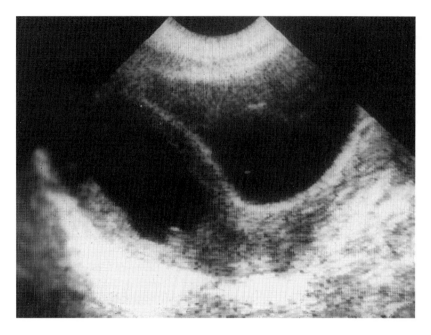

Use the above figure to answer question 3.011.

3.011 This image MOST likely represents a(n):
   A. blighted ovum
   B. complete spontaneous abortion
   C. ectopic pregnancy
   D. normal intrauterine gestation, but too early to detect the fetal pole

A is correct.
Although the yolk sac is seen inferiorly, no fetal pole is visible, leading to the conclusion that this is probably a blighted ovum. The sac is too large to be too early to see a fetal pole. The amount of fluid seen here is much greater than would be expected after a complete spontaneous abortion, and the presence of an intrauterine yolk sac appears to preclude this being an ectopic pregnancy.

3.012 In a patient with a complete spontaneous abortion, the MOST likely finding is a(n):
   A. empty gestational sac with no evidence of decidua
   B. embryo with no evidence of a heartbeat
   C. complex mass in the cul-de-sac
   D. empty uterus with a decidual reaction

D is correct.
In a complete spontaneous abortion, all products of conception are passed, although some fluid may remain in the sac. Decidual reaction may persist for 2 weeks. If a non-viable embryo is present, this is considered to be fetal demise or a missed abortion.

3.013 A patient < 20 weeks LMP presents with a closed cervical os and a distorted gestational sac in a low uterine position. This MOST likely represents a(n):
   A. blighted ovum
   B. complete spontaneous abortion
   C. threatened abortion
   D. inevitable abortion

C is correct.
Although a distorted gestational sac low in the uterus is a serious concern, it does not inevitably lead to abortion. If profuse bleeding and a dilated os are not present, and if there is a positive fetal heartbeat, a majority (84–98%) may progress to term. The presence of a subchorionic hemorrhage with placental separation from the uterine wall is an additional indicator of a poor prognosis.

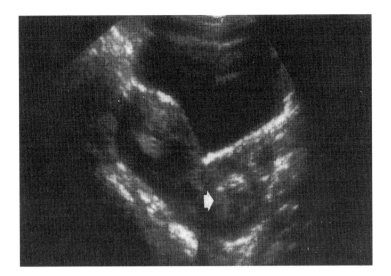

Use the above figure to answer question 3.014.

3.014 This MOST likely represents a(n):
    A. threatened abortion
    B. incomplete abortion
    C. missed abortion
    D. inevitable abortion

D is correct.
An inevitable abortion may appear as a misshapen gestational sac very low in the uterine neck or cervix. In this case, the presence of a complex mass in the cervix is an indication that abortion is inevitable. A threatened abortion may appear lower in the uterus than normal, but never in the neck or cervix. If a heartbeat is discerned in a threatened abortion, the prognosis is usually good. An incomplete abortion usually presents with abnormal echogenic or anechoic areas within the enlarged uterus and increased endometrial echoes, with or without a gestational sac. This may lead to a septic uterus, wherein shadowing from gas-producing organisms may be seen.

3.015 With respect to ectopic pregnancies, which of the following is TRUE?
A. an adnexal mass can usually be palpated
B. implantation in the interstitial portion of the tube is a common occurrence
C. cornual ectopic pregnancies may have dangerous prognoses
D. ectopic pregnancies cannot be carried past the first trimester

C is correct.
Cornual ectopic pregnancies are not often seen and are difficult to diagnose, as they are easily mistaken for intrauterine implantations. Due to the high vascularity of this area, catastrophic bleeding may occur with rupture. An adnexal mass may be present in approximately half of all ectopic pregnancies. The mass should be examined for the presence of cardiac motion or a yolk sac. In a tubal ectopic pregnancy, the interstitial portion, that part of the tube contained within the cornu of the uterus, is the least likely site of implantation. The ampullary portion of the tube is the more usual site for ectopic pregnancies. Abdominal ectopics have been known to be carried to term, with the first indication of problems at the onset of labor. If an ectopic pregnancy is suspected, it is important to examine the cul-de-sac for the presence of fluid or a complex mass, the hepatorenal space for the presence of free fluid, and the uterine endometrium for the presence of a gestational sac.

Second and third trimesters

3.016 When measuring the ventricular system of the fetal head, the MOST accurate level to use is the:
A. frontal horn
B. lateral ventricle parallel to the falx
C. lateral ventricular atrium
D. cisterna magna

C is correct.
Although the lateral ventricular wall ratio (specifically, the distance from the midline echo to the lateral wall of the lateral ventricle divided by the distance from the midline echo to the inner table of the lateral skull) is most frequently used to assess ventricular normalcy, there is some question as to whether the linear echo usually designated 'lateral ventricle wall' is indeed that structure or, in fact, a vascular structure. Recent investigations indicate that a more confident measure may be made at the widest diameter of the atrium, through the choroid plexus and perpendicular to the long axis of the atrium rather than perpendicular to the falx.

3.017 Measurement of the cerebellum is BEST made at the level of the:
A. thalamus, hippocampus, midbrain, cavum septum pellucidum
B. vermis, midbrain, cisterna magna
C. sphenoid, temporal bone, pituitary stalk
D. foramen magnum, pons, fourth ventricle

B is correct.
Choice A includes structures at the level of the biparietal diameter and head circumference measurements, and choices C and D include structures at the base of the brain.

3.018 In a sagittal sonogram of a second-trimester fetal spine, the 'railroad-track' appearance represents the:
   A. spinal canal and spinous processes
   B. vertebral body and posterior lamina
   C. vertebral body and spinous process
   D. posterior laminae and pedicles

B and C are correct.
Depending on the angle of insonation, the outermost 'track' represents either the midsagittal spinous process or the more lateral lamina structure. The spinal canal is visualized as a long thin anechoic region in the middle of the railroad tracks.

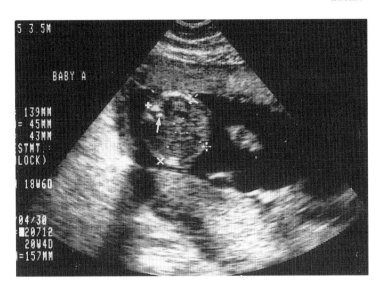

Use the above figure to answer question 3.019.

3.019 In this image of the transverse fetal spine, the arrow is pointing to the:
   A. spinous process
   B. posterior lamina
   C. transverse process
   D. vertebral body

D is correct.
Whereas it is important to obtain coronal or sagittal views of the spine and to visualize the intact skin covering the cranial and lumbosacral areas, it is also important to view the spine throughout its length in a transverse plane. Splaying of the dorsal processes is best evaluated in this manner. In a sagittal view, splaying may be hidden by the angle of the scan.

3.020 A percentage of fetal blood from the IVC is shunted from the:
   A. left atrium to right atrium
   B. right atrium to left atrium
   C. IVC to the ductus venosus
   D. right atrium to the ductus arteriosus

B is correct.
Prior to entering the fetal heart, some of the blood from the umbilical vein is shunted to the IVC via the ductus venosus, bypassing the fetal liver. From the IVC, blood enters the right atrium, where 60% is shunted to the left atrium via the foramen ovale due to the slightly higher right atrial pressure, and 40% enters the right ventricle; 90% of the blood that enters the right ventricle is then shunted from the pulmonary artery to the aorta through the ductus arteriosus, bypassing the fetal lungs.

3.021 Visualization of a four-chambered heart within the fetal thorax enables determination of the:
    A. position of the heart and size of the ventricles
    B. patency of the atrioventricular valves
    C. patency of the ventriculoarterial valves
    D. relative sizes of the aortic root and left atrium

A and B are correct.
Cardiac structures are best seen at 20–34 weeks. The apex of the heart should point to the same side as the stomach. The four-chambered view also allows determination of atrioventricular concordance, and integrity of the atrial and ventricular septa. The left atrium can be recognized by the flap of the foramen ovale. It is the chamber closest to the fetal spine, and should be contiguous with the left ventricle (which has papillary muscles, but no moderator band). Visualization of the pulmonary and aortic valves, and the aortic root, requires cephalad angling of the transducer whereas a 90° turn is required to evaluate the ratio of the aortic root to the left atrium.

3.022 Which of the following is NOT a reason to perform sonography of the fetal thorax?
    A. to visualize symmetric clavicles
    B. to evaluate lecithin:sphingomyelin (L:S) ratio
    C. to evaluate the integrity of the diaphragm
    D. to determine cardiac position

B is correct.
The L:S ratio is a clinical means of evaluating lung maturity. Sonographic assessment of the fetal thorax provides information regarding lung anatomy and may rule out pleural effusion. The echogenicity of the lung is similar to that of the liver early in gestation and greater than that of the liver later on. It has been thought that placental grading correlated with lung maturity, but this is no longer believed to be true.

3.023 With respect to ultrasound of the fetal thorax, which of the following is TRUE?
    A. the diaphragm presents as a linear echoic band
    B. increased thickness of skin at the ventral aspect of the thorax usually indicates pathology
    C. the long axis of the fetal heart is usually perpendicular to the long axis of the body
    D. visualization of some fluid in the pleural space is normal

C is correct.
The fetal heart is much more perpendicular to the chest wall (closer to the transverse axis of the thorax) than is the adult heart. The diaphragm is appears as a linear **hypoechoic** band. It is evaluated coronally for evidence of fetal breathing and to rule out herniation of abdominal structures into the thorax. Often, maternal hormones cause transient thickening of breast tissue in both male and female fetuses. Although a small amount of pericardial fluid may be normal, no fluid should be seen in the pleural space.

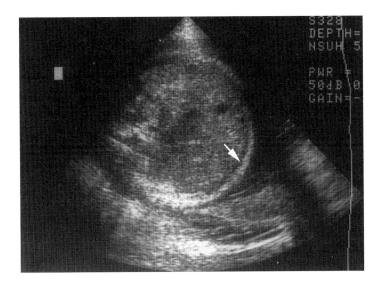

Use the above figure to answer question 3.024.

3.024 In this image, the hypoechoic area indicated by the arrow is MOST likely:
  A. fetal ascites
  B. the subcutaneous abdominal muscle layer
  C. fetal pleural effusion
  D. the diaphragm

B is correct.
Subcutaneous abdominal muscle layers appear hypoechoic. At times, this area may be prominent and give the appearance of 'pseudo-ascites'. True fetal ascites appears as an anechoic mass **surrounding** and lying between fetal abdominal structures. Fetal pleural effusion is always an indicator of fetal distress and/or pathology.

3.025 An 11-week-old fetus presents with an outpouching from the anterior abdominal wall into the base of the umbilical cord. This is MOST likely to be:
  A. gastroschisis
  B. omphalocele
  C. normal herniation of the fetal gut
  D. peristalsis

C is correct.
At around 9 weeks, the small bowel herniates into the proximal umbilical cord, where it grows and loops around the superior mesenteric artery (SMA). Further looping occurs at the end of 12 weeks as it returns to the abdomen. Thus, midline anterior abdominal wall defects cannot be diagnosed prior to 14 weeks. Gastroschisis is not an accurate alternative as it does not involve the umbilical cord, but rather consists of an abdominal wall defect, usually to the right of the umbilicus. Peristalsis is the normal muscular movement of the digestive tract.

3.026 With regard to bowel, which of the following is TRUE?

   A. peristalsis can be seen in the small bowel, but not in the large bowel
   B. peristalsis can be seen in the large bowel, but not in the small bowel
   C. the presence of echogenic meconium in the small bowel is normal early in the second trimester
   D. the presence of echogenic meconium in the small bowel is a sign of fetal distress

A and C are correct.

Early in the second trimester, meconium in the small bowel causes an echogenic appearance. The meconium is gradually propelled to the colon, where it remains as a normal finding. However, meconium in the amniotic fluid late in the third trimester (meconium staining) or in the fetal abdomen outside the bowel (meconium peritonitis) suggests a pathologic condition such as bowel perforation. The sterile meconium in the peritoneal cavity causes an intense reaction leading to calcification. Further irritation may cause fibrotic reaction and formation of meconium pseudocysts, seen as complex calcified masses. These may be confused with teratomas or calcified neuroblastomas. With ultrasound, it is difficult to distinguish an amniotic bleed or meconium staining in the amnion from normal amnion containing vernix.

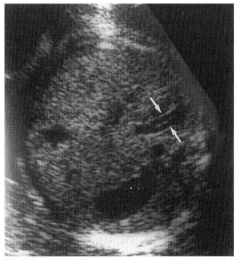

Use the above figure to answer question 3.027.

3.027 In this image, which of the following fetal structures are enclosed by the arrows?

   A. kidney
   B. adrenal gland
   C. stomach
   D. gallbladder

B is correct.

Fetal adrenal glands are proportionately much larger than adult adrenals and may sometimes be mistaken for the fetal kidney. Fetal adrenal length is around one-half to two-thirds of fetal renal length. (The circumference of each fetal kidney is around one-third the abdominal circumference.) The fetal adrenal gland consists of a hyperechoic medulla and a thicker hypoechoic outer cortex. The relatively thick fetal zone of the cortex atrophies within the first 3–12 months after birth. Fetal adrenals can be imaged after 30 weeks of gestation. The kidneys are seen as early as 15 weeks. Before that time, they are undeveloped.

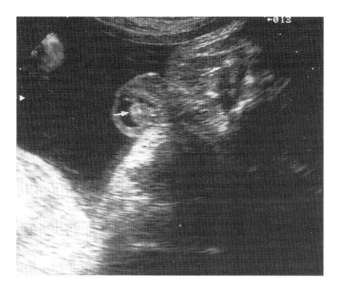

Use the figure above to answer question 3.028.

3.028 In this image, the arrow is pointing to the:
   A. scrotum
   B. labia
   C. testes
   D. choroid plexus

C is correct.
The testes are usually sonographically visible within the scrotum after 32 weeks. It is not unusual, in the late third trimester, to see fluid in the scrotum surrounding the testicles either unilaterally, as here, or bilaterally. This is called a hydrocele and is not a sign of pathology. It usually has no apparent cause and the fluid disappears prior to birth or shortly thereafter.

3.029 Which of the following structures is MOST likely to be visible in the fetal pelvis?
   A. iliac crests and sacrum
   B. hypoechoic gluteal muscles
   C. ischium and pubis
   D. bladder

All are correct.
Although the fetal pelvis is small, the pelvic bones, muscles and bladder can be routinely imaged. When the bladder is full of urine, it extends into the fetal abdomen. Similarly, if ovarian cysts are seen, they extend into the abdomen due to the small pelvic size.

3.030 It is important to assess the fetal bladder on every examination. Which of the following statements is TRUE?
   A. if the bladder appears distended, then pathology is indicated
   B. a full bladder means that at least one kidney is functioning
   C. the fetus voids approximately once per hour
   D. if the bladder is not seen, pathology is indicated

B and C are correct.
The bladder may appear distended without the presence of pathology. Rescanning after 20–40 min will confirm whether voiding has taken place, an indication of normal bladder function. Similarly, if the bladder is not seen, it may be because the fetus has recently voided. Another scan should be taken after 30 min to visualize the bladder.

3.031 Transvaginally, it is possible to assess all fetal long bones, and fingers and toes, by _____ weeks of gestation.
  A. 10
  B. 14
  C. 18
  D. 22

B is correct.
This is possible at ± 16 weeks transabdominally. The anteriorly located long bone should be used for dating, as it produces less artifactual distortion in measurement. The posteriorly located limb may appear shorter than it is due to its position. However, this can be compensated for by including the distal epiphyses in the measurement of the posteriorly lying femur; both should be evaluated to assure growth symmetry. Any apparently abnormal flexion or position of the limb may indicate a pathology and should be noted. If the fetal foot is visualized in the same plane as the tibia or fibula, this may indicate the presence of a clubfoot deformity.

3.032 Normal fetal limb assessment is MOST likely to be characterized by which of the following?
  A. the femur slightly larger than the humerus from week 16 onwards
  B. the fibula (lateral shaft) thicker than the tibia
  C. the distal radius and ulna ending at the same point
  D. the foot and the tibia seen in the same imaging plane

A and C are correct.
Linear transducers provide less distortion and a larger field of view for all obstetric measurements, thereby producing a more accurate measurement, particularly for anteriorly located structures. A linear transducer is generally better than a sector transducer for obtaining the most accurate measurements.

3.033 Evaluation of fetal lie and position is important because:
  A. the heart cannot be seen unless the fetus is in a vertex position
  B. it is necessary in the determination of situs
  C. if the fetus is in a breech position, it may render measurement of the femur difficult
  D. different organs may best be seen with varying fetal positions

B, C and D are correct.
In second-trimester gestations, the heart may be imaged with the fetus in any position, but it is best seen with the fetal spine lying posterior, or to the mother's right or left side. In late gestations, spine and rib shadowing make imaging the heart difficult if the fetus is not lying on its back. The fetus can change position up to the time of delivery.

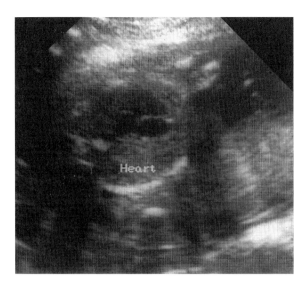

Use the above diagram to answer question 3.034.

3.034 In this image, the chamber lying CLOSEST to the fetal spine is the:
  A. left atrium
  B. right atrium
  C. left ventricle
  D. right ventricle

A is correct.
The left atrium lies closest to the fetal spine and receives the four pulmonary veins. The right atrium receives the IVC and SVC. The papillary muscles are seen in the left ventricle, which is the more posteroinferolateral ventricular chamber. The right ventricle, the most anteriorly situated chamber of the heart, contains the moderator band. It is also important to remember that the heart lies more perpendicular in the fetal thorax than it is in adults. Thus, in the fetus, the vertex points more anteriorly, with the plane of the axis perpendicular to the chest wall. The sonographer should always confirm that the apex of the heart points towards the fetal stomach.

Placenta, umbilical cord and fetal Doppler

3.035 Deoxygenated fetal blood enters the placenta through the:
  A. umbilical vein
  B. umbilical artery
  C. spiral artery
  D. uterine artery

B is correct.
Deoxygenated fetal blood enters the placenta via the two umbilical arteries, which spiral around the single, larger, umbilical vein. The fetal vessels branch into the chorionic villi within the placenta. Oxygenated maternal blood from spiral arterioles at the base of the placenta is delivered into the intervillous space, bathing the chorionic villi. Oxygen and nutrients are exchanged across the villous membranes. Oxygenated blood is then carried to the fetus via the umbilical vein.

3.036 The trophoblast, the outermost layer of cells of the blastocyst surrounding the fluid-filled cavity and inner cell mass, produces which of the following hormones?
   A. human chorionic gonadotropin (hCG)
   B. progestrone
   C. estrogen
   D. gonadotropic-stimulating hormone

A is correct.
hCG causes the corpus luteum to persist and become the corpus luteum of pregnancy. This assures continued secretion of progesterone from the corpus luteum. Progesterone prevents the endometrial lining from sloughing off and allows the trophoblast to develop into the placenta.

3.037 The chorionic membrane of the placenta is formed from the:
   A. syncytiotrophoblast
   B. decidua capsularis
   C. mesenchyme
   D. cytotrophoblast

C and D are correct.
The trophoblast differentiates into two layers: an inner cytotrophoblast and an outer syncytiotrophoblast. The cytotrophoblast surrounds the mesenchyme, a loose network of cells that forms the extraembryonic coelom and body stalk. The cytotrophoblast and mesenchyme eventually become the outer surface and villi of the chorion. The syncytiotrophoblast forms the chorion laeve and frondosum. The villi of the chorion frondosum at the point of implantation proliferate, eventually forming the placenta, whereas those of the chorion laeve normally disappear. The decidua are formed from uterine tissue.

3.038 Regarding placental structure and location, which of the following is usually TRUE?
   A. the placenta is 3–4 cm in thickness
   B. the chorionic plate meets the basal plate at the edge of the placenta
   C. placental attachment to the myometrium may be anywhere in the uterus
   D. maternal draining veins are located at the lateral margins of the placenta

B and C are correct.
The placenta is normally 1.5–4 cm in thickness (some consider 5 cm the upper limit of normal). In general, the larger the basal plate, the thinner the placenta; thickness increases with placental age. The maternal draining veins lie posterior to the placenta and are readily seen on ultrasound. The hypoechoic draining veins should not be included when measuring placental thickness nor should they be mistaken for other possible hypoechoic masses, such as retroplacental hemorrhage.

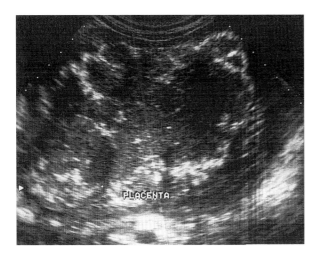

Use the above figure to answer question 3.039.

3.039 In this image, the placenta is MOST likely to have a:
  A. chorioangioma
  B. subplacental hematoma
  C. Breus' mole
  D. grade III placenta

D is correct.
A grade 0 placenta is homogeneous with a smooth chorionic plate. A grade I placenta contains some echogenic areas (representing calcifications) randomly dispersed in the placental mass and has subtle indentations on the chorionic plate. A grade II placenta has echogenicities along the basal plate and more indentations on the chorionic plate. A grade III placenta contains many echogenicities, is lobulated and may contain anechoic areas in the central portion of one or more lobes. It is important to remember that not every term pregnancy contains a grade III placenta. Many normal placentas are only grade II or even I at term. Breus' mole (also called 'massive subchorionic thrombosis') is a type of large placental hematoma on the placental surface which bulges into the amniotic cavity. The prognosis for this lesion is uncertain.

3.040 A single umbilical artery (SUA) may indicate anomalies in which of the following systems?
  A. cardiac
  B. gastrointestinal
  C. central nervous (CNS)
  D. renal

A, C and D are correct.
Renal anomalies are most commonly associated with SUA, although cardiac and CNS anomalies have also been found. The two umbilical arteries are longer than the vein, and all are longer than the amnion casing, resulting in the normal twisting of these vessels within the cord. The vessels within the amnion are surrounded by Wharton's jelly. Vasa praevia occurs when fetal vessels run intramembranously across the internal os. These vessels may tear during delivery and may be seen sonographically. In contrast, portions of the cord length seen in a dilated cervix inferior to the presenting part of the fetus are referred to as 'prolapsed'.

3.041 Placental abruption, or premature separation of all or part of the placenta from the uterine wall, is MOST likely to present with which of the following?
  A. an apparently normal placenta
  B. a retroplacental mass of varying echogenicity
  C. an apparently thickened placenta
  D. a subchorionic or intraplacental hypoechoic mass

All are correct.
Placental abruption may present with all or some of these findings. External bleeding may or may not be present as early as the first trimester. It is important not to confuse the retroplacental complex of maternal veins with retroplacental hemorrhage or abruption.

3.042 Placenta previa is MOST likely to present in association with which of the following?
  A. increased maternal age, increased parity or previous abortion
  B. second trimester bleeding
  C. a distance from presenting part to maternal sacrum or maternal bladder < 1.5 cm
  D. a placenta extending to and covering the fundus

A is correct.
Placenta previa usually presents with bleeding in the late third trimester and may be associated with abruption at that time. If the presenting part to maternal sacrum or bladder measurement is < 1.5 cm, it is unlikely there will be anterior or posterior previa. This, however, does not rule out lateral previa. Usually, if the placenta extends to the fundus, then no previa is present; however, a thin flat placenta may extend from the fundus to the area of the os, or an accessory lobe may cover or impinge on the os. Thus, if possible, the os should also be evaluated. It is important that the bladder is not too full to avoid artifactual elongation of the cervix presenting a false appearance of previa.

3.043 A chorioangioma is BEST described as:
  A. a malignant lesion
  B. the most common tumor of the placenta
  C. usually associated with other structural placental pathology
  D. not always sonographically detectable

B and D are correct.
This benign lesion is usually located on the fetal surface of the placenta. Its appearance may vary from homogeneous and solid to hypoechoic with cystic or solid components. It may be mistaken for venous lakes or organizing blood clots, or appear as normal placental tissue. Chorio-angioma may not be associated with other **structural** abnormalities of the placenta, but there may be vascular shunting leading to fetal hydrops, low birth weight, etc.

3.044 A grade III placenta prior to term (according to Grannum *et al.*):
  A. may be associated with hyaline membrane disease
  B. indicates a lecithin:sphingomyelin ratio ≥ 2
  C. is directly related to fetal lung maturity
  D. may be associated with intrauterine growth retardation (IUGR), maternal hypertension and fetal distress

A and D are correct.
Previously, placental grading according to the amount and location of placental calcifications was thought to be directly related to lung maturity (L:S ratio); however, it is now considered that the two may be related, but that one is not predictive of the other.

3.045 By the start of the second trimester, the spiral arterioles have become dilated due to the action of the cytotrophoblast. This is MOST likely to be seen on ultrasound evaluation of the uterine or arcuate arteries through a Doppler waveform characterized by:
  A. high resistance with increased diastolic flow
  B. high resistance with decreased diastolic flow
  C. low resistance with increased diastolic flow
  D. low resistance with decreased diastolic flow

C is correct.
A low-resistance system allows for increased diastolic flow with lower blood pressure. A diastolic flow that is decreased and/or a systolic:diastolic ratio that is increased indicates constricted vessels with increased resistance to flow. The results of such increased resistance may be preeclampsia and intrauterine growth retardation.

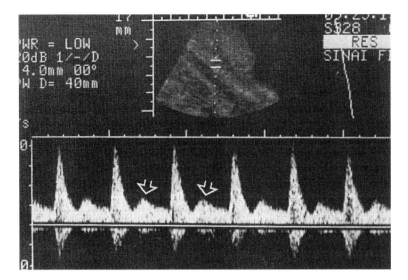

Use the above figure to answer question 3.046.

3.046 This pulsed-wave Doppler waveform from a maternal uterine artery shows early diastolic notching (arrows). This notch is MOST likely:
- A. normal if present throughout pregnancy
- B. normal if seen after 20 weeks of gestation
- C. normal if seen before 16 weeks, but abnormal after 20 weeks of gestation
- D. abnormal throughout pregnancy

C is correct.

The notch is normally seen prior to 16 weeks of gestation and in non-pregnant women where the early diastolic resistance is high. After 20 weeks, however, there is normally a decrease in vascular impedance in the placenta, which allows higher diastolic flow in the uterine artery. The persistence of the early diastolic notch, therefore, corresponds to elevated placental vascular resistance in early diastole. This indicates that there is inadequate placental nutrition and oxygenation. The persistent notch can be seen in association with maternal hypertension and intrauterine growth retardation.

Assessment of gestational age

3.047 Of the following, the MOST accurate means of dating a gestation is with a(n):
  A. gestational sac measurement at 5 weeks transvaginally
  B. yolk sac seen in a 2.0-cm gestational sac
  C. crown-rump length (CRL) measurement at 7 weeks
  D. head circumference (HC) measurement at 20 weeks

C is correct.
The accuracy of the CRL measurement is good for ± 4 days. The gestational sac can usually be seen transvaginally at 5 weeks LMP, although the accuracy of its size as a predictor of gestational age is only valid for up to ± 2 weeks. Visualization of a yolk sac is a good indicator of a viable pregnancy if seen in a gestational sac ≥ 2.0 cm. It is not, however, a specific predictor of gestational age. HC is considered more accurate than the biparietal diameter (BPD) in the second and third trimesters, having an accuracy of ± 1 week (BPD is ± 2 weeks).

3.048 Regarding BPD measurement as a predictor of gestational age, which of the following is TRUE?
  A. BPD is more accurate than femur length in the late third trimester
  B. BPD is more accurate than femur length in the second trimester
  C. BPD is can be routinely measured from 12 weeks of gestation
  D. BPD is more accurate than HC in the second trimester

B and C are correct.
After 33 weeks of gestation (± 2.2 weeks), femur length is considered more accurate than the BPD. Head circumference is also fairly accurate, but not always easily obtained in very late pregnancies. It should also be remembered that, as the pregnancy progresses, individual genetic factors (parental height, etc.) have greater significance and affect fetal measurements more than in early pregnancy.

3.049 Regarding femur length measurement, it is BEST to include the:
  A. osseous femoral diaphysis (shaft) only
  B. osseous femoral diaphysis including the femoral head
  C. osseous femoral diaphysis including the epiphyses
  D. osseous femoral diaphysis including the condyles

A is correct.
The femoral shaft measurement appears to be the least affected by position or molding. The accuracy of predictability is limited to genetic factors, and correlates with fetal age and crown–heel length at birth. Use of a linear transducer gives the most accurate measurement. The femoral shaft should be perpendicular to the beam.

3.050 The largest transverse section of the abdomen is MOST likely found at the location of the:
  A. umbilicus
  B. confluence of the umbilical and portal veins
  C. stomach and the umbilical vein
  D. fetal kidneys

B and C are correct.
The abdominal circumference (AC) measurement should be taken at the largest transverse section of the abdomen, and taken when both the stomach and umbilical vein are imaged, as the umbilical vein enters the portal vein. (Also adequate is when a short segment of the umbilical vein is seen one-third of the way into the center of the abdomen along with the stomach.) If the kidneys are seen in this view or if the umbilical vein is seen close to the anterior abdominal wall, then the plane of view is oblique rather than truly transverse and should therefore not be used.

3.051 Regarding the transverse HC measurement, which of the following is TRUE? It is:
   A. usually considered to be less accurate than the BPD
   B. usually considered to be more accurate than the BPD
   C. taken at the level of the cerebral peduncles
   D. taken at the level of the cerebellum

B is correct.
The transverse HC measurement is not affected by intrinsic or pressure-induced change in head shape which can render the BPD measurement of fetal age erroneous. HC should be taken at the same level as the BPD – at the level of the cavum septa pellucida, thalami and interhemispheric fissure –at the outer margins of the cranium.

3.052 Of the following measurements, which is the BEST for estimating fetal age if a BPD or HC are not obtainable?
   A. binocular distance (outer orbital diameter)
   B. interocular distance
   C. diameter of the atrium of the lateral ventricle
   D. cerebellar length

A is correct.
The binocular distance from outer edge to outer edge of the ocular globes is a fairly good parameter for estimation of fetal age in the absence of a good BPD or HC, albeit less accurate than either. The atrial diameter is a measurement of lateral ventricular size and not specifically related to fetal age. Cerebellar size is not a function of age.

3.053 The cephalic index (CI) is:
   A. OFD ÷ BPD × 100
   B. BPD ÷ OFD × 100
   C. brachycephalic if < 70%
   D. brachycephalic if > 90%

B and D are correct.
The fetal head is considered dolichocephalic if the CI is < 70%. If the fetal head is either brachy- or dolichocephalic, it is customary to rely more on the HC rather than the BPD measurement, as a very narrow or wide BPD may give an erroneous estimate of fetal age.

Complications: Intrauterine growth retardation

3.054 Fetal lung maturity (L:S ratio ≥ 2) is:
   A. sonographically assessable with placental grading
   B. sonographically assessable with HC measurements
   C. sonographically assessable through lung echogenicity
   D. not sonographically assessable

D is correct.
Although placental grading was previously thought to be a means of evaluating lung maturity, it has since been shown that there is little causal relationship between them. The L:S ratio is determined by amniocentesis.

3.055 Intrauterine growth retardation (IUGR) is BEST defined as a fetus that is:
   A. below the 10th percentile in weight
   B. usually associated with maternal hypertension
   C. at high risk of perinatal morbidity
   D. none of the above

C is correct.
Although fetuses below the 10th percentile should be evaluated for IUGR (as is defined by some clinicians), these may simply be small fetuses due to genetic/population factors. Estimated fetal weight below the 5th percentile (2 SD < mean weight) is now accepted by most as growth retardation. Maternal hypertension, smoking, drug abuse, disease, genetic and chromosomal factors, and chronic fetal infections are among the many causes of IUGR. Perinatal morbidity is increased and fetal mortality increased six- to tenfold when associated with IUGR.

3.056 Which of the following finding(s) is(are) MOST likely to be associated with IUGR?

    A. oligohydramnios
    B. polyhydramnios
    C. 'prematurely mature' placenta
    D. a markedly decreased HC:AC ratio

A and C are correct.

Remember that a finding of oligohydramnios is not specific for IUGR, as the condition may have other causes, such as premature rupture of membranes (PROM). However, decreased amniotic fluid (largest vertical pocket < 2–3 cm) in a fetus that is < 5th to 10th percentile with a grade III placenta before week 36 of gestation is suggestive of IUGR. Asymmetric IUGR shows a markedly increased HC:AC ratio whereas, with symmetric IUGR, this ratio is not altered from the norm, although both measurements are reduced. Asymmetric IUGR manifests later than the symmetric form (after 28 weeks), and fetal head growth is usually normal until late in pregnancy due to preferential blood flow to the brain. A decreased HC:AC ratio is more suggestive of a macrosomic fetus.

3.057 Complete each of the following statements with the correct word or phrase.

    A. In IUGR, the estimated fetal weight is usually _____ below the norm
    B. An abnormal ponderal index is seen in fetuses with an FL in the 90th percentile and an AC below the 10th percentile. These fetuses will have growth retardation even if their _____ is normal
    C. Computation of a baseline fetal heart rate and changes in response to fetal movement is known as a _____
    D. A score of _____ on a biophysical profile is normal

A. 2 SD
B. EFW
C. non-stress test. This test is also affected by the periodicity of certain fetal biophysical functions, such as breathing and movement.
D. 8. Note that this is a better predictor of normal than abnormal, as many low scores can be accounted for by the normal periodicity of fetal functions.

3.058 Fetal Doppler studies of IUGR have shown that increased vascular resistance in the fetal aorta and umbilical artery is MOST likely to be associated with:

    A. decreased resistance in the internal carotid artery (ICA)
    B. increased resistance in the ICA
    C. asymmetric IUGR
    D. symmetric IUGR

A and C are correct.

Increased vascular resistance in the fetal aorta and umbilical artery, characterized by decreased or absent diastolic flow, produces an increased systolic:diastolic ratio. This is accompanied by decreased resistance in the fetal ICA, leading to the brain-, heart- and adrenal-sparing phenomenon at the expense of the extremities seen in asymmetric IUGR. Markedly increased systolic:diastolic ratios in the fetal aorta or umbilical artery are associated with increased perinatal morbidity and mortality. It should be remembered, however, that other factors may affect the Doppler waveform, such as the site of sampling. The highest resistances are recorded in the cord nearest to the abdominal insertion site. Fetal breathing, pharmacologic agents and technical factors may also affect Doppler signals.

Complications: Multiple gestations

3.059 Regarding multiple gestations, when two ova are fertilized, this is BEST described as:
    A. monozygotic (MZ) twinning
    B. dizygotic (DZ) twinning
    C. monochorionic (MC) and monoamniotic (MA) twinning
    D. monochorionic and diamniotic (DA) twinning

B is correct.
DZ twinning results from two separate fertilized ova, each of which becomes a blastocyst with a separate implantation site. Each embryo has its own chorion, amnion and placenta. In contrast, MZ twinning may produce one of several combinations, depending upon when the single fertilized ovum was split. DZ twins are indistinguishable by ultrasound from dichorionic (DC) DA twins of MZ origin.

3.060 Conjoined twins only occur in a monozygotic situation and when the fertilized ovum splits at _____days.
    A. 1–4
    B. 5–9
    C. 10–13
    D. > 13

D is correct.
If the ovum splits within 3 days of gestation, a DC, DA gestation is produced, with each embryo in its own amniotic sac and its own placenta (although the placentas may be fused and appear to be one). If the split occurs later, but before the end of the first week of gestation, an MC, DA gestation results. Each embryo has its own amniotic sac, but both share a single chorion with a single placenta. If the split occurs between 10–13 days, the result is MC, MA with one placenta. After 13 days, splitting is incomplete and results in conjoined twins. A variable percentage of MC twin pregnancies are reported to have vascular anastomoses between the circulations of the two fetuses which may cause a group of syndromes, such as twin-to-twin transfusion (TTT), which may affect the morbidity and mortality of MC twins. DC placentas, even when fused, do not appear to develop such vascular anastomoses.

3.061 Which of the following complications is NOT generally associated with multiple gestations?
    A. intrauterine growth retardation of one or both twins
    B. increased incidence of preeclampsia
    C. increased third-trimester bleeding
    D. post-term labor

D is correct.
Premature labor is one of the most common complications of a multiple pregnancy (52% are delivered before term). IUGR may occur as a result of TTT in MC twins, causing hydrops of the other twin. Interestingly, it is usually the twin with IUGR who has the better prognosis, rather than the hydropic twin. Increased bleeding may be due to placenta previa, abruption or velamentous insertion of the cord, which may occur in multiple gestations. Other complications are maternal gestational hypertension and an increased incidence of developmental abnormalities, especially in MA pregnancies. According to Berman, a normal fetus with a Turner's syndrome twin is the most common discordant genetic defect in MZ twins.

3.062 In a twin pregnancy, visualization of a septum > 1.0 mm in width is MOST likely to represent which type of twinning?
    A. dichorionic (DC)
    B. monochorionic (MC)
    C. diamniotic (DA)
    D. monoamniotic (MA)

A is correct.
All DC pregnancies must also be DA, with each twin surrounded by its own amnion and chorion. Therefore, the septum between them is made up of four layers of fetal membrane, leading to a thicker appearance on ultrasound. MC, DA membranes are usually thin and only visualized in short segments. MC, MA twins have the poorest prognosis. Note that the presence of a membrane within the gravid uterus does not always indicate a multiple pregnancy. Another type of membranous structure seen in singleton pregnancies is amnion separated from the chorion either prior to its normal fusion, or abnormally as part of an amniotic band or amniotic sheet.

Complications: Maternal illness

3.063 Which of the following is MOST likely to be found in the fetuses of diabetic mothers?
    A. intrauterine growth retardation
    B. macrosomia
    C. skeletal and CNS abnormalities
    D. cardiac, renal and gastrointestinal abnormalities

All are correct.
Diabetes mellitus as well as maternal hypertension, collagen–vascular disease, renal disease and malnutrition may all compromise fetal oxygenation and lead to IUGR. Doppler umbilical findings, specifically, the persistence of a notch at the beginning of the diastolic phase after 24 weeks of gestation and/or persistently elevated uterine artery systolic: diastolic ratios, are indicators of inadequate nutrition and oxygenation. Anomalies in fetuses of diabetic mothers have an estimated incidence of 3–6%. Diabetes may lead to macrosomia due to increased sugar entering the fetal circulation, and may cause maturational delays and disrupt organogenesis in the fetus. Some anomalies associated with diabetic mothers are neural tube defects, ventricular septal defects, ureteral duplication, duodenal atresia and single umbilical artery. Gestational diabetes has similar effects on the fetus except that its later onset during gestation prevents the disruption of organogenesis.

3.064 Which of the following is the MOST likely risk factor for gestational diabetes?
    A. family history of diabetes
    B. previous baby with congenital anomalies
    C. history of Rh isoimmunization
    D. there are no risk factors

A and B are correct.
Other risk factors are previous stillbirth or a previous macrosomic infant. Although diabetes mellitus may be a cause of Rh isoimmunization, the converse is not true. Gestational diabetes generally has the same effect on the developing fetus as pregestational diabetes; however, the later the onset of the condition, the less likely is the fetus to be affected during organogenesis.

3.065 The presence of hypertension in the second or third trimester is MOST likely to increase the risk of:

  A. fetal hydrops
  B. intrauterine growth retardation
  C. placental abruption
  D. toxemia
  E. polyhydramnios

B, C and D are correct.

Toxemia of pregnancy occurs in the third trimester and has two stages – preeclampsia (the development of hypertension with proteinuria and/or maternal edema) and eclampsia (characterized by maternal convulsions). Immunologic, hormonal and nutritional factors are thought to be responsible. Toxemia is also associated with fetal distress and fetal demise.

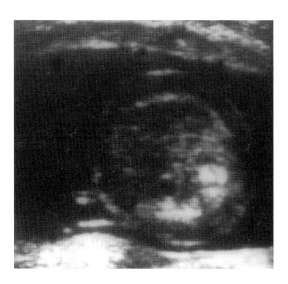

Use the above figure to answer question 3.066.

3.066 The sonographic finding in this image is MOST likely be associated with which of the following?

  A. viral infection
  B. Rh isoimmunization
  C. sickle cell anemia
  D. malnutrition

A and B are correct.

Fetal hydrops, with its associated findings of polyhydramnios, fetal ascites, pericardial effusion, fetal anasarca (seen here), thick placenta and cardiomegaly, may be caused by many non-immunologic conditions and viral infections. These include obstructive vascular problems, pulmonary disease, neoplasms and chromosomal anomalies. Sickle cell anemia and malnutrition are more likely to produce low birth-weight fetuses.

Antepartum

3.067 Which of the following is LEAST likely to be associated with preterm labor?

    A. twinning
    B. premature rupture of membranes (PROM)
    C. cervical cerclage
    D. Rh isoimmunization

C is correct.
Premature labor is the spontaneous onset of obvious regular contractions between weeks 20 and 37 of pregnancy, and is the most common complication of multiple gestation. It may be due to overdistention of the uterus with subsequent contractions, or because of premature rupture of the membranes from excess pressure. It may also have no specific underlying cause. Rh isoimmunization is often associated with polyhydramnios, which may lead to preterm labor for similar reasons. Cervical cerclage is a procedure for securing the cervix when the inner os is incompetent (width of opened cervix > 2.0 cm). An incompetent cervix usually occurs early in the second trimester. It is painless and bloodless, and tends to recur with each pregnancy.

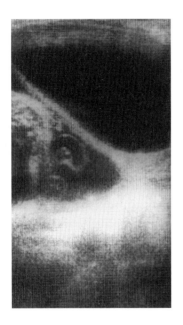

Use the above figure to answer question 3.068.

3.068 This image is MOST likely to represent which of the following conditions?

    A. occult vessels
    B. dilated cervix
    C. vasa praevia
    D. frank prolapse

C is correct.
The cervix in this image is > 2.5 cm and appears to be intact. Segments of cord are seen between the cervix and the presenting part (vasa praevia), but not within the cervical canal (frank prolapse) or on either side of the presenting part (occult). Rembember that segments of cord within the amniotic fluid cannot always be visualized on 2-D ultrasound.

Fetal therapy

3.069 Regarding fetal blood sampling (PUBS), it is BEST to involve percutaneous sampling of the:
- A. umbilical vein near the cord insertion at the placenta
- B. umbilical vein near the cord insertion at the umbilicus
- C. unbilical artery near the cord insertion at the placenta
- D. umbilical vessels within the placenta

A is correct.
Fetal blood sampling is performed to verify amniocentesis or chorionic villus sampling results, or for rapid chromosomal diagnosis. Samples obtained from the placenta, although easier to obtain, may be mixed with maternal blood.

Postpartum

3.070 Which of the following is NOT a cause of postpartum hemorrhage?
- A. puerperal infection
- B. delayed uterine involution
- C. retained products of conception
- D. prolonged labor

A is correct.
Puerperal infection in itself is not a cause of postpartum hemorrhage, but prolonged labor is a cause of puerperal infection and may be associated with postpartum hemorrhage. Deep anesthesia may prevent timely postpartum involution (contraction) of the uterus. Thus, the blood vessels that are normally occluded by the muscle contractions remain open and are prone to bleed. Retained products of conception (i.e. placental tissue) cause the uterine cavity to remain enlarged with bleeding at the placental site. An overdistended uterus as well as placental implantation abnormalities may also cause postpartum hemorrhage.

3.071 Which of the following is MOST likely to cause postpartum infection?
- A. obesity
- B. increased age or parity
- C. prolonged labor
- D. delayed uterine involution

C is correct.
Other possible causes of postpartum infection are poor hygiene, use of invasive monitoring devices, anemia, vaginitis, toxemia and retention of placental parts. Obesity and increased age or parity may be contributing factors in puerperal ovarian vein thrombophlebitis.

3.072 Among the sonographic findings on examination of a postpartum uterus is an echogenic mass within the uterine myometrium, with hyperechoic areas and acoustic shadowing. This MOST likely represents which of the following?
- A. endometritis
- B. puerperal ovarian vein thrombophlebitis
- C. bladder-flap hematoma
- D. Cesarean-section abscess

D is correct.
Although endometritis may also exhibit shadowing due to gas formation, it normally does not present as an echogenic mass, but rather as an anechoic region separating the two walls of the endometrial cavity. Thrombophlebitis appears as an anechoic or hypoechoic mass in the upper retroperitoneal cavity – not the uterus – and may exhibit Doppler blood flow. A bladder-flap hematoma may appear as a complex, poorly marginated, mass and may have internal septations. It is located between the uterus and maternal bladder. Bladder-flap hematoma and abscess may appear similar on ultrasound, and clinical correlation may be required to distinguish them.

Amniotic fluid and lung maturity

3.073 Increased frequency of polyhydramnios (or hydramnios) is MOST often associated with which of the following conditions?
   A. maternal diabetes mellitus
   B. decreased fetal fluid consumption
   C. bilateral renal agenesis
   D. intrauterine growth retardation

A and B are correct.
The majority of cases of polyhydramnios are idiopathic (60%), with 20% due to fetal causes (CNS or gastrointestinal anomalies) and 20% due to maternal causes. Increased fluid volume produces uterine stretching and enlargement that may lead to preterm labor. Although it is commonly thought that hydramnios is common in twin gestations, only 5–10% of twin pregnancies have this finding. When present, it appears to be associated with an increased fetal mortality rate, especially when it develops acutely. Bilateral renal agenesis typically causes severe oligohydramnios.

3.074 Prolonged severe oligohydramnios is MOST likely to lead to which of the following conditions?
   A. hip dislocation
   B. pulmonary hypoplasia
   C. post-term pregnancy
   D. single umbilical artery (SUA)

A and B are correct.
The most serious condition caused by increased pressure on the fetus is pulmonary hypoplasia. In general, the lower the fluid volume, the worse the prognosis. Infants with oligohydramnios-induced pulmonary hypoplasia usually die of severe asphyxiation shortly after birth. Post-term pregnancy (with decreased fetal urine production) may be a **cause** of oligohydramnios, not a result. Other possible causes are placental insufficiency associated with IUGR, resulting in fetal hypoxia which, in turn, leads to redistribution of fetal blood away from the kidneys. (PROM may lead to oligohydramnios, but is more associated with post-term pregnancy in conjunction with IUGR and placental insufficiency than with preterm labor.) SUA may be associated with urinary anomalies such as bilateral renal agenesis and posterior urethral valves, but these may be a cause of oligohydramnios, not a result. Umbilical cord compression (causing fetal asphyxia) may be a result of oligohydramnios.

3.075 The gold standard for evaluating fetal lung maturity is the L:S ratio. An L:S ratio ≥ 2.0 indicates lung maturity. Estimation of fetal lung maturity with ultrasound is MOST accurate using which of the following parameters?
  A. determination of accurate fetal age
  B. measurement of thorax circumference
  C. biparietal diameter of 9.2 cm
  D. placental calcification grading

A is correct.
This allows elective delivery after 38 weeks with virtually no risk or, alternatively, accurate L:S ratio determination by amniocentesis. Some studies suggest that a BPD > 9.2 cm (at ± 38 weeks) is evidence of fetal lung maturity in the absence of diabetes. However, there is no evidence that all BPDs of 9.2 cm are at least 38 weeks of gestational age. It is the number of weeks that is important, not the BPD. After 38 weeks, lung maturity is certain. Placental grading is not an indicator of lung maturity. Many fetuses with grade III placentas have L:S ratios < 2.0. In addition, only 10–20% of pregnancies attain a grade III placenta by term.

Genetic studies

3.076 The likelihood that maternal serum screening using alpha-fetoprotein, unconjugated estriol and hCG will detect cases of Down syndrome is:
  A. 20%
  B. 40%
  C. 60%
  D. 80%

C is correct.
If tested only for AFP, the likelihood falls to 20%. Maternal serum screening is one means of diagnosing chromosomal disorders prenatally. Advanced maternal age, family history and ethnicity are all risk factors. Other techniques used in prenatal genetic testing are chorionic villus testing, fetal blood and tissue sampling, and amniocentesis.

3.077 Amniotic-fluid testing (amniocentesis) under ultrasound guidance has become a standard procedure and is MOST likely to be performed:
  A. at 24–26 weeks of gestation
  B. to assess karyotype or for DNA extraction
  C. to monitor the fetus during the procedure
  D. to monitor the bilirubin concentration in amniotic fluid

B, C and D are correct.
Generally, amniocentesis is performed at 16–18 weeks of gestation, when sufficient fluid is present, to allow 24 ml of fluid to be removed with ease. Also, if an anomaly is found, there is time to elect termination. Continual ultrasound monitoring during amniocentesis ensures that the fetus does not get in the way of the needle and allows assessment of problems if fluid is not immediately obtained. The severity of hemolytic disease (Rh isoimmunization) is related to the bilirubin level, which can be evaluated by serial amniocenteses. PUBS may be performed instead of amniocentesis in these cases.

3.078 Ultrasound-guided chorionic villus sampling is MOST likely to be performed:
  A. at 10–12 weeks of gestation
  B. either transabdominally or transcervically
  C. because CVS risk is comparable to that of amniocentesis
  D. to evaluate trophoblast tissue

All are correct.
CVS allows for earlier genetic testing than is possible with amniocentesis. Thus, if termination is necessary, it can be performed earlier and with greater safety. Ultrasound also allows for determination of a viable fetus prior to the procedure.

3.079 Chromosomal disorders occur in approximately
_____ of live births.
   A. 0.5%
   B. 5%
   C. 15%
   D. 50%

A is correct.
The incidence associated with spontaneous abortions is closer to 50%. These chromosomal abnormalities include abnormalities of total chromosome number (for example, Turner's syndrome and a trisomy such as Down syndrome), genetic defects in single genes where total chromosomal number is normal (for example, cystic fibrosis), and polygenic or multifactorial disorders (1%; including cleft lip, cardiac abnormalities, omphalocele, renal agenesis and thalassemia), which carry a risk of recurrence and higher familial relationship.

Fetal demise

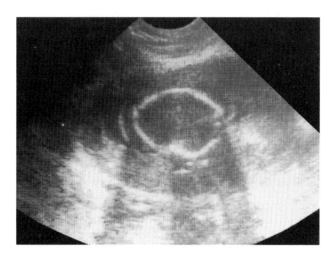

Use the above figure to answer question 3.080.

3.080 In this image, the fetal head is MOST likely exhibiting which of the following?
   A. Spalding's sign
   B. holoprosencephaly
   C. choroid plexus cyst
   D. scalp edema

A and D are correct.
Sonographic findings associated with fetal demise include Spalding's sign (overlapping skull bones), absence of umbilical cord pulsations, oligohydramnios and fetal edema. However, these signs alone are not definitive for fetal demise. Only the absence of a fetal heartbeat, and cord pulsations with a lack of fetal movement, should be considered definitive. The other, secondary, signs become apparent 12–48 hours after fetal death.

3.081 The term 'fetus papyraceus' refers to a condition wherein the fetus:
- A. is reabsorbed, leaving no detectable sign
- B. lacks normal bone structure
- C. lacks red blood cells, rendering it white as paper
- D. dies, but persists as a flattened structure with bones

D is correct.
The fetus is rather like a fossilized remnant. Often, in twin gestations, one twin remains viable whereas the other, which may have been viable at 10 weeks, dies spontaneously at a later date and persists only as an amorphous or flattened structure. Twin demise earlier in pregnancy is usually reabsorbed.

Fetal abnormalities

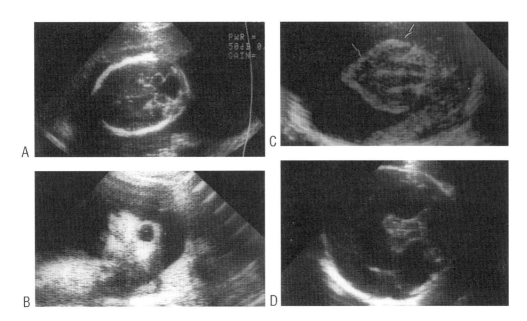

Use the above figures to answer question 3.082.

3.082 The conditions shown in A–D, respectively, are:
- A. _____
- B. _____
- C. _____
- D. _____

- A. Dandy–Walker malformation, which is characterized by the fourth-ventricle defect of a retrocerebellar cyst communicating with the fourth ventricle (which becomes greatly enlarged through a defect of the cerebellar vermis). There may be accompanying degrees of hydrocephalus.
- B. Anencephaly, which is sonographically diagnosed when the cranial vault above the level of the orbits cannot be seen after 14 weeks (if the fetal lie is not obstructive). The cerebral hemispheres are also absent.
- C. Hydranencephaly, in which the cystic replacement of the cerebral hemispheres is thought to be due to congenital infection or occlusion of the internal carotid arteries.
- D. Holoprosencephaly, which describes a variety of midline cranial and facial abnormalities, such as absent falx. There is a single common ventricle.

3.083 The MOST accurate method for evaluating hydrocephalus is to measure the diameter of the:
   A. atrium of the lateral ventricle through the choroid plexus
   B. superior lateral ventricle from the falx to the lateral margin of the ventricle
   C. fourth ventricle at the level of the cerebellum
   D. frontal horns at the level of the thalami

A is correct.
The more superior plane, where the 'lateral ventricle' is parallel to the falx cerebri, may not accurately portray the true margin of the ventricle but may, in fact, represent a venous structure. The atrial measurement, taken slightly inferiorly and towards the occipital horn, is more accurate. In early hydrocephalus, the shrunken choroid plexus is anteriorly displaced, indicating detachment from the medial wall of the ventricle.

3.084 Sonographic evaluation of bilateral cleft lip and palate may be made as early as _____ weeks.
   A. 10
   B. 14
   C. 18
   D. 22

B is correct.
Although complete cleft lip and palate may be seen early in the second trimester, unilateral or incomplete cleft lip may be more difficult to visualize, depending on the plane of view. The incomplete cleft may not sufficiently involve the integrity of the nose to be easily recognized. The median cleft lip is a rare form that may be associated with holoprosencephaly and other intracranial anomalies. Clefts are generally subtle and may be difficult to diagnose by ultrasound. Diagnosis is also highly dependent on fetal position.

3.085 Hypotelorism can BEST be described as a condition which includes:
   A. a severely sloping forehead
   B. fetal orbits that are too close together [decreased interorbital diameter (IOD)]
   C. a possible association with an abnormal nose
   D. a severely reduced fetal chin

B and C are correct.
In fact, a decreased IOD is the definition of hypotelorism, which may be indicative of a severe brain malformation. It is most commonly associated with holoprosencephaly. The orbital defects range from mild to severe (cyclopia), and include cataracts. In more severe hypotelorism, the nose is abnormal, having a tubular appearance as it protrudes from the face from above the single orbit. In a less severe form, the nose may be positioned normally, but may have only one nostril. In a fetus with a sloping forehead, microcephaly is suspected (although microcephaly is a **biometric**, not a morphologic, diagnosis); a reduced chin may indicate micrognathia. Both are associated with multiple congenital abnormalities.

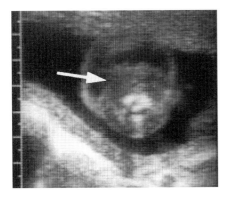

Use the above figure to answer question 3.086.

3.086 In this image, the structure indicated by the arrow is MOST likely a:
   A. cystic hygroma
   B. cephalocele
   C. teratoma
   D. choroid plexus cyst

A is correct.
Congenital malformations of the lymphatic system, appearing as single or multilocular fluid-filled cavities, are known as cystic hygromas. These cystic masses most often appear on the neck (posterolaterally) due to failure of lymphatic drainage into the jugular venous system. This may result in generalized fetal edema (hydrops fetalis). Although cystic hygromas are associated with Turner's syndrome, they often appear in fetuses without that pathology. Cephaloceles are protrusions of the meninges (and sometimes the brain) through cranial defects. Choroid plexus cysts usually resolve by the end of the second trimester, although some association with trisomy 18 has been observed. A teratoma may appear to be both cystic and solid.

3.087 A complex mass appearing on either side of the fetal neck is MOST likely to be a:
   A. meningomyelocele
   B. cephalocele
   C. teratoma
   D. choroid plexus cyst

C is correct.
Although most teratomas are sacrococcygeal, they may be found throughout the body. Depending on the size and position of the teratoma, it may compress the upper airway and proximal esophagus, producing hydramnios. Teratomas are usually benign neoplasms that do not recur. They are usually solid with some cystic areas. Depending on their location, they may prevent normal vaginal delivery. Teratomas can be resected after birth, but there may be other associated anomalies. A meningomyelocele may appear as a complex mass, but it is located along the dorsal aspect of the fetus and protrudes from the spine. Cystic hygromas are common in the neck area and may be bilateral. They are predominantly cystic or loculated.

3.088 A spinal defect containing meninges and neural tissue is MOST likely to be a:
- A. cephalocele
- B. spina bifida
- C. meningocele
- D. meningomyelocele

D is correct.

Cephaloceles are protrusions of brain and/or meninges through a defect in the cranium. Spina bifida is the failure of fusion of the two halves of the vertebral arch. When meninges protrude through this spinal defect, it is called a meningocele and, when accompanied by neural tissue, is termed a meningomyelocele. Neural tube defects are associated with elevated maternal serum alpha-fetoprotein.

3.089 The 'lemon sign' and 'banana sign' are MOST usually associated with which of the following?
- A. Arnold–Chiari malformation
- B. Dandy–Walker malformation
- C. spina bifida
- D. indigestion

A and C are correct.

These 'signs' refer to malformations of the front of the cranium and cerebellum, respectively. The malformations reflect displacement of tissue from the cerebellar vermis into the upper cervical spinal canal. Most cases are associated with open spina bifida and hydrocephalus. It is thought that the open lower spine with its meningeal protrusions causes the brain matter to be drawn into the spinal canal which, in turn, may result in the deformity at the front of the fetal head.

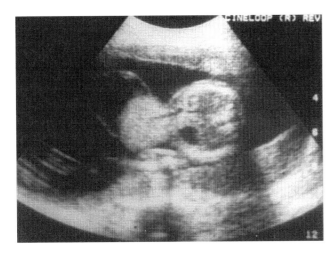

Use the above figure to answer question 3.090.

3.090 This image MOST likely shows which of the following defects?
   A. gastroschisis
   B. omphalocele
   C. ectopia cordis
   D. bladder exstrophy

B is correct.
All are defects in the anterior wall of the fetus. Omphaloceles involve herniation of viscera into the base of the umbilical cord through a midline abdominal wall defect. Cord can be seen in the omphalocele surrounded by amniotic membrane. Normal rotation of the embryonic bowel occurs in the base of the umbilical cord between weeks 6 and 10 and, therefore, the diagnosis of omphalocele cannot be made prior to ± 12 weeks. With gastroschisis, the umbilicus is normal and the defect occurs usually to the right of the cord insertion. Herniated viscera are seen floating in the amniotic fluid. Gastroschisis is associated with gastrointestinal anomalies whereas omphaloceles have a high association with these and other assorted anomalies. Ectopia cordis involves a lower sternum defect with the heart lying anterior to the chest wall, and may be associated with amniotic band syndrome, omphalocele and other deformities. It is important to differentiate bladder exstrophy from urachal cyst, a less common deformity, seen as a cystic mass between the bladder and umbilicus along the anterior abdominal wall.

3.091 Which of the following anomalies involving abdominal wall defects is MOST usually incompatible with life?
   A. omphalocele
   B. gastroschisis
   C. bladder exstrophy
   D. limb–body wall complex

D is correct.
This complex involves anomalies of the abdomen and thorax as well as cranial, facial and limb deformities. It may be associated with amniotic band syndrome. Herniated viscera and skeletal defects are seen on sonography.

3.092 Sonographic visualization of a fluid-filled mass behind the left atrium and ventricle in the lower thorax MOST likely represents:
A. cystic adenomatoid formation
B. congenital diaphragmatic hernia (CDH)
C. pleural effusion
D. cardiac effusion

B is correct.
CDH causes a mass effect manifested by lung compression and reduction of functional lung tissue. If this occurs prior to 16 weeks, pulmonary hypoplasia results. Even if viscera are not seen in the thorax, absence of a stomach in the abdomen, a small AC and polyhydramnios are suggestive of CDH. Cystic adenomatoid formation is usually unilateral and seen as a single large, or several smaller, cystic areas lateral to the heart. Multiple tiny cysts may appear as a single solid homogeneously echogenic structure. A single small cyst in the lungs may also be a bronchiogenic cyst. Pleural effusion generally follows the contour of the lungs and diaphragm, and appears lateral to the heart; pericardial effusion does not usually appear posterior to the atria. Fetal pleural effusion is abnormal at any time and may indicate hydrops fetalis, chest mass or other abnormalities. If large, a pleural effusion may cause flattening of the diaphragm and bulging of the chest wall.

3.093 A well-circumscribed echogenic mass in the fetal thorax is MOST likely to represent which of the following conditions?
A. congenital diaphragmatic hernia
B. pulmonary sequestration
C. cystic adenomatoid malformation
D. normal lung tissue

B and C are correct.
One type of cystic adenomatoid malformation consists of multiple tiny cystic masses which cannot be sonographically resolved and, thus, appear as a single echogenic mass. Pulmonary sequestration also appears as an echogenic mass in the thorax, usually on the left. Extralobar pulmonary sequestration, the type most commonly seen prenatally, consists of a mass of ectopic lung tissue enveloped by is own pleura, fed and drained by non-pulmonary (i.e. systemic) vessels, and lacking communication with the normal bronchial tree.

3.094 Oligohydramnios after week 16 of gestation is MOST likely to indicate which of the following?
A. unilateral renal agenesis
B. bilateral renal agenesis
C. multicystic dysplastic kidney
D. cystic renal dysplasia

B and D are correct.
Unilateral renal agenesis is more common than the bilateral form, but may be difficult to identify on sonography, as the fetal adrenal gland is large and may be mistaken for the missing kidney. The contralateral kidney tends to be large and, as long as one kidney has function, fluid is present in the fetal bladder in normal amounts. As multicystic dysplastic kidney is usually unilateral, fluid amounts are normal. Cystic renal dysplasia, however, which is secondary to an early genitourinary tract obstruction such as posterior urethral valves, is usually accompanied by significant oligohydramnios due to the obstruction. Prior to week 16, the lack of fetal input to the amniotic fluid is masked by the placental component.

3.095 The most common renal tumor of neonates which is MOST likely to be seen prenatally is the:
- A. nephroma
- B. Wilms' tumor
- C. neuroblastoma
- D. cryptorchidism

A is correct.

The usually benign congenital mesoblastic nephroma or hamartoma may present as a unilateral echogenic mass, often with hydramnios. Wilms' tumor, which may be bilateral and malignant, has not been sono-graphically demonstrated antenatally. Neuro-blastoma is the most common abnormality of the fetal adrenal glands. It may appear as a complex or mixed mass, and calcification may be present. It has been associated with hydrops fetalis. Cryptorchidism, or undescended testicles, may be suspected sonographically by failure to see the testicles within the fetal scrotum. It is usually isolated, but may be part of the prune-belly triad.

3.096 The genital anomaly MOST likely to be detected sonographically *in utero* is:
- A. hydrometrocolpos
- B. hydroureter
- C. ovarian cyst
- D. Müllerian duct cyst

A is correct.

The incidence of hydrometrocolpos slightly exceeds that of ovarian cysts well into adolescence. The enlarged uterus may then compress the urinary tract and cause hydronephrosis or hydroureter. In female fetuses, the Müllerian ducts develop into the Fallopian tubes and uterus.

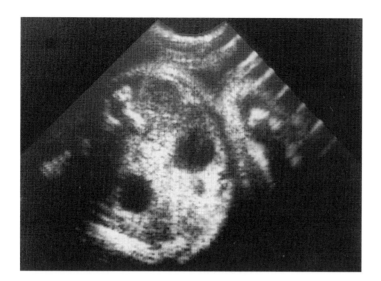

Use the above figure to answer question 3.097.

3.097 In this image, the MOST likely condition being visualized is:

    A. duodenal atresia
    B. esophageal atresia
    C. jejunal obstruction
    D. meconium ileus

A is correct.
Duodenal atresia is the most common congenital gastrointestinal tract obstruction, and may be seen prenatally. It is characterized on sonography by the double-bubble sign of distended stomach and proximal duodenum, and is seen with polyhydramnios. However, the double-bubble sign is not specific for duodenal atresia and appears with annular pancreas, duodenal stenosis, volvulus and other gastrointestinal obstructions. Duodenal atresia is associated with other anomalies, including congenital heart disease, and renal, spinal and other gastrointestinal anomalies. Esophageal atresia may be sonographically demonstrated by the presence of polyhydramnios and non-detection of the fetal stomach after 14–15 weeks of gestation.

3.098 Sonographic visualization of multiple interconnecting anechoic structures in the lower abdomen is MOST likely to represent:
   A. Caroli's disease
   B. jejunal obstruction
   C. esophageal atresia
   D. meconium ileus

B is correct.

Jejunal or ileal obstruction may be demonstrated on sonography by multiple interconnecting distended bowel loops, depending on the level of obstruction. With higher levels of obstruction, the incidence of polyhydramnios increases. If intestinal perforation occurs, fetal ascites and meconium peritonitis may be visualized. Meconium ileus, or obstruction of the distal small bowel by meconium, occurs in conjunction with cystic fibrosis. It may be seen sonographically as abnormal areas of increased echogenicity in the fetal abdomen, small bowel dilatation and polyhydramnios. These are, of course, non-specific findings. Caroli's disease is ectasia of the biliary ducts and, if present, is seen in the liver.

3.099 Which of the following is MOST likely to be sonographically visualized as a fluid-filled mass in the right upper quadrant of the fetal abdomen?
   A. congenital duplication cyst
   B. choledochal cyst
   C. urachal cyst
   D. ascites

A, B and D are correct.

Urachal cysts occur near the mid-ventral abdominal wall rather than in the upper right quadrant. Duplication cysts may be found anywhere along the gastrointestinal tract. A choledochal cyst is a localized dilatation of the biliary system, usually the comon bile duct. Ascites, which is always abnormal in the fetus, sometimes collects between the two leaves of unfused omentum, which may then appear as an upper abdominal cyst.

3.100 A fetus with sonographic findings of a narrow thorax, curved and shortened long bones, and a cloverleaf skull is MOST likely to have which of the following?
   A. osteogenesis imperfecta
   B. achondroplasia
   C. VACTERL syndrome
   D. thanatophoric dysplasia

D is correct.

Thanatophoric dysplasia is the most common lethal skeletal dysplasia. It is frequently accompanyied by hydrocephaly and polyhydramnios. Achondroplasia is the most common non-lethal skeletal dysplasia. The bones of the hands and feet are short, and the head is large. Osteogenesis imperfecta is a collagen disorder with varying degrees of hypomineralization of the skeleton. Sonographic depiction of shortened or bowed long bones or ribs, or multiple fractures *in utero* may suggest the condition. VACTERL comprises the following: vertebral anomalies; anal atresia; cardiac anomalies; tracheoesophageal fistula; renal anomalies; and limb dysplasia. The presence of at least three of these is required to make this diagnosis.

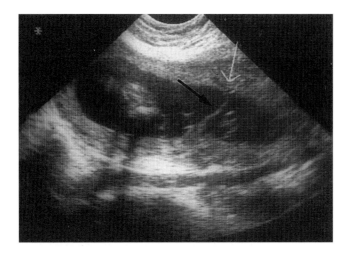

Use the above figure to answer question 3.101.

3.101 In this image of a 28-week-old singleton gestation, the black arrow is MOST likely pointing to a(n):
    A. amniotic band
    B. chorionic band
    C. placental band
    D. jazz band

A is correct.
Amniotic band syndrome can be associated with limb amputation, facial clefts and body wall defects. It is suggested that amniotic bands are formed by rupture of the amnion, leading to transient oligohydramnios and subsequent entanglement of fetal tissue with the fibrous bands attached to the chorionic side of the amnion. The fetus may also adhere to the exposed chorion, producing further maldevelopment. Deformities produced by amniotic bands are generally asymmetric.

3.102 Which of the following congenital cardiac anomalies CANNOT be diagnosed *in utero*?
    A. Ebstein's anomaly
    B. tetralogy of Fallot
    C. transposition of the great arteries
    D. patent ductus arteriosus

D is correct.
The ductus arteriosus is a vascular connection between the aorta and pulmonary artery. It should be patent in the fetus, as its purpose is to shunt a proportion of fetal blood from the pulmonary to the systemic circulation while bypassing the lungs. It is only an anomaly if it remains open after birth. The foramen ovale serves the same purpose. The ductus venosus allows some of the blood returning to the fetus in the umbilical vein to bypass the liver circulation by entering the hepatic veins or IVC directly.

3.103 Which of the following cardiac anomalies is MOST likely to be associated with intrauterine heart failure?
A. double-outlet right ventricle
B. hypoplastic left heart syndrome
C. transposition of the great arteries
D. large ventricular septal defect (VSD)

B is correct.
Sonography shows a very small left ventricle accompanied by mitral and/or aortic atresia. The ascending aorta is also hypoplastic. The right side of the heart is usually enlarged and the fetus may or may not be hydropic. The prognosis is always poor. A double-outlet right ventricle is usually accompanied by one or more septal defects which serve to accommodate adequate fetal circulation. Transposition of the great arteries is often associated with other cardiac anomalies, such as VSD, pulmonary stenosis and coarctation of the aorta. There are two types – corrected and uncorrected – and neither causes hemodynamic distress to the fetus. After birth, however, uncorrected transposition must be surgically altered to adjust to the neonatal circulation. VSD is the most common form of congenital heart disease in the fetus. Large VSDs are easily visualized and usually do not result in hemodynamic compromise *in utero*.

3.104 Which of the following is MOST likely to be an antenatal sonographic clue to the presence of Marfan syndrome?
A. enlarged limbs due to edema
B. asymmetric limb hypertrophy
C. visceromegaly
D. very long extremity bones

D is correct.
Fetuses with long extremity bones may be at risk for this autosomal-dominant connective tissue disorder. Patients with this disorder are typically very tall and thin, with cardiac anomalies such as dilated/aneurysmal aortic root and holosystolic mitral valve prolapse.

3.105 Failure of the common atrioventricular (AV) valve orifice to separate into mitral and tricuspid valves is MOST likely to be part of which of the following?
A. tetralogy of Fallot
B. endocardial cushion defect
C. hypoplastic heart syndrome
D. Ebstein's anomaly

B is correct.
Defects in the AV valves, primum portion of the atrial septum and membranous portion of the ventricular septum give rise to endocardial cushion defects. These defects are usually seen together as they develop from the same embryological tissue at the same time, and are classified as either complete or partial. A complete AV canal has a large AV defect with a common septal leaflet. The interatrial septum may be absent and there may be a large membranous VSD. This is often associated with Down syndrome. A partial AV canal usually has a small primum defect and a VSD of varying size, and a cleft mitral valve.

3.106 Sonographic findings of a thickened nuchal fold, shortened femurs and hypoplasia of the middle phalanx of the fifth digit are MOST likely to be associated with which of the following conditions?
    A. trisomy 13
    B. trisomy 18
    C. trisomy 21 (Down syndrome)
    D. Turner's syndrome

C is correct.
These are all chromosomal defects. Down syndrome is also associated with cardiac anomalies such as endocardial cushion defects. If the nuchal fold is > 5 mm in an unextended fetal neck, the fetus should be carefully evaluated for other signs. Although the nuchal fold sign has been reported in association with other anomalies and in normal fetuses, its presence on ultrasound is ample reason for amniocentesis. This is especially true for mothers < 35 years old, who are less likely to undergo routine amniocentesis than are older mothers.

3.107 A fetus presenting with holoprosencephaly, midline facial abnormalities, polydactyly, congenital heart disease, omphalocele and polycystic kidneys is MOST likely to have which of the following chromosomal disorders?
    A. trisomy 13
    B. trisomy 18
    C. trisomy 21 (Down syndrome)
    D. Turner's syndrome

A is correct.
Trisomy 13 is a rare disorder usually with a poor prognosis. Trisomy 18 is a relatively common collection of defects also associated with a poor prognosis. These include polyhydramnios, IUGR, clubfoot, clenched hand, and cardiac, renal and other abnormalities leading to fetal distress and premature delivery. Turner's syndrome is characterized by short stature, sexual infantilism and a short neck in female fetuses, often with associated cystic hygromas (often called 'webbed neck'). Renal anomalies are common. When cystic hygromas arise in places other than the neck, they are usually not chromosomally related.

3.108 Sonographic findings of oligohydramnios, absent kidneys, IUGR and pulmonary hypoplasia are MOST consistent with:
    A. Meckel–Gruber syndrome
    B. Potter's syndrome
    C. amniotic band syndrome
    D. prune-belly syndrome

B is correct.
Potter's syndrome is the result of severe oligohydramnios due to impaired renal function, which may be due to one of several causes, including UPJ, but not necessarily absent kidneys. Death due to pulmonary insufficiency may occur after birth. Meckel–Gruber syndrome is characterized by occipital encephalocele, bilateral multicystic dysplastic kidneys and polydactyly. It is fatal at birth due to pulmonary hypoplasia secondary to oligohydramnios which, in turn, is secondary to renal failure. Also associated are cleft lip, micrognathia and short limbs. There is a 25% risk of recurrence as it is autosomal-recessive. Amniotic alpha-fetoprotein is usually elevated in this syndrome. Prune-belly (Eagle–Barrett) syndrome comprises abdominal muscle deficiency, urinary tract dilatation and cryptorchidism; and may include a wide variety of other defects such as cardiac anomalies, patent urachus in conjunction with urethral atresia, and limb deformities resulting from oligohydramnios. Familial recurrence has been noted.

Coexisting disorders

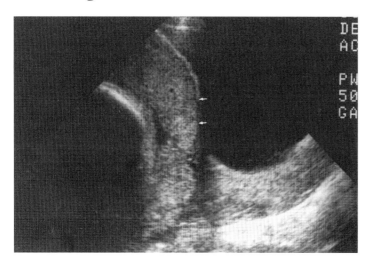

Use the above figure to answer question 3.109.

3.109 In this image, the placenta MOST likely demonstrates which of the following conditions?
    A. placenta membranacea
    B. abruptio placentae
    C. placenta previa
    D. placenta percreta

C and D are correct.
There are varying degrees of abnormal placental invasion of the uterine wall, from the mildest (accreta) to percreta, which extends to the serosal surface and may even invade adjacent organs. Placenta accreta is generally used to describe all three conditions. In this instance, along with complete placenta previa, placental tissue appears to extend to the external uterine wall in several places. There is a high association with placenta previa, which has the same predisposing conditions. Abruptio placentae refers to premature separation of the placenta from the uterine wall, and is associated with pain and bleeding. On sonography, there is evidence of subplacental hemorrhage, which may have varied appearances, although intrauterine hematoma is not always present. Small hematomas may be asymptomatic, but larger ones may result in fetal hypoxia with subsequent growth retardation and death. Trauma, maternal hypertension, age, parity, uterine anomalies, cocaine abuse and toxemia have been reported among the causative factors.

3.110 An allantoic duct cyst is MOST likely to be associated with which of the following intrauterine structures?
    A. umbilical cord
    B. placenta
    C. fetal urinary tract
    D. fetal gastrointestinal tract

A is correct.
These cysts may occur anywhere along the cord and may be associated with a patent urachus. True cysts are small and may be remnants of the allantois. False cysts are the result of liquefaction of Wharton's jelly, which coats the cord, and may be very large. Both types of cyst are usually asymptomatic.

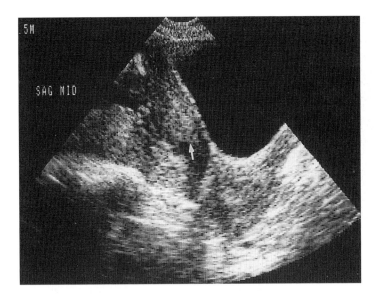

Use the above figure to answer question 3.111.

3.111 In this image, the arrow is MOST likely pointing to which of the following?
- A. contraction
- B. fibroid
- C. placenta previa
- D. placental abruption

A is correct.

In this case, anterior and posterior contractions of the lower uterine segment, lying just above the internal cervical os, have caused the placenta to appear to be partially covering the os. Uterine contractions occur throughout pregnancy (Braxton Hicks contractions), becoming more frequent and intense as parturition is approached. A contraction usually disappears after 20–30 min. Also, a contraction extends inwards towards the uterine cavity whereas a myoma usually extends towards the outer margin of the uterus. Demonstration of the linear choroid plate is sufficient to differentiate placental tissue from a fibroid or contraction.

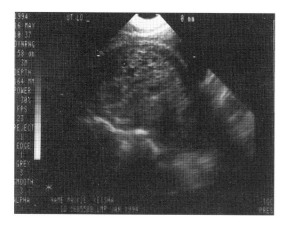

Use the above figure to answer question 3.112.

3.112 In this image, the uterus is MOST likely to contain a(n):

    A. myoma
    B. degenerating myoma
    C. Breus' mole
    D. hydatidiform mole

D is correct.

Although degenerating myomas may contain numerous cystic areas which may mimic trophoblastic changes, increased β-hCG levels confirm the hydatid nature of the mass. On sonography, the hydatidiform mole may appear anechoic or have areas of variable echogenicity. The mole generally occupies all or most of the endometrial cavity and resembles placental tissue with multiple anechoic areas (vesicular appearance). Breus' mole, which is a large hematoma of the placenta, is not related to the hydatidiform mole.

3.113 The maternal cystic mass that is MOST likely to be seen during pregnancy is the:

    A. dermoid cyst
    B. corpus luteum cyst
    C. mesenteric cyst
    D. theca-lutein cyst

B is correct.

Cystic masses during pregnancy are usually ovarian in origin, although fluid-filled bowel and hydrosalpinx are difficult to distinguish from ovarian masses. Large cystic masses, especially pedunculated dermoid cysts, are prone to torsion and may rupture. Corpus luteum cysts of pregnancy are usually unilateral, singleton and 2–6 cm in diameter, although they may reach 10 cm in diameter. Dermoid cysts may be cystic or complex masses and are also referred to as 'benign cystic teratomas'; however, dermoid tumors contain only ectodermal elements (hair, teeth and sebaceous material) whereas teratomas contain ecto-, meso- and endodermal elements. If rupture occurs, as it may during delivery, it can cause chemical peritonitis. Mesenteric cysts are rare pelvic masses that may be septate. Theca-lutein cysts are associated with gestational trophoblastic disease, multiple gestations or ovarian hyperstimulation, and are usually bilateral and multilocular. As they are caused by increased levels of hCG, they tend to regress when hCG levels return to normal.

3.114 Choriocarcinoma is MOST likely to develop from a(n):

    A. hydatidiform mole
    B. normal term pregnancy
    C. ectopic pregnancy
    D. spontaneous abortion

All are correct.

Choriocarcinoma is the most malignant form of gestational trophoblastic disease, but only 50% of these neoplasms develop from a hydatidiform mole. The other 50% develop from the other three choices listed. The patient presents with persistent vaginal bleeding after evacuation of uterine contents, persistently elevated β-hCG is and/or theca-lutein cysts. The lungs and vagina are common sites of metastases. First-trimester Doppler evaluation of the uterine artery in a patient with gestational trophoblastic neoplasm shows increased flow compared with that associated with myomas or normal pregnancy.

3.115 During pregnancy, demonstration of a solid fusiform or rounded structure near the maternal bladder with a central echogenic area is MOST likely to be:

    A. a wandering spleen
    B. a pelvic kidney
    C. appendicitis
    D. colonic cancer

B is correct.

This is the most likely structure to be found of that description if careful examination of the renal fossae determines that one of the kidneys is not in its proper location. However, appendicitis and colonic cancer cannot be ruled out without careful examination of the clinical symptoms. On occasions, the early signs and symptoms of these diseases may be attributed to the pregnancy and thus ignored. When sonographically demonstrated, appendicitis more often appears as a tubular complex mass, and the finding of an appendicolith with acoustic shadowing within the mass is pathognomonic. Colonic cancer often mimics the appearance of a pelvic kidney. Wandering spleen may cause pain early in pregnancy, but its homogeneous appearance is unlikely to be confused with that of the kidney.

GYNECOLOGY

Normal pelvic anatomy

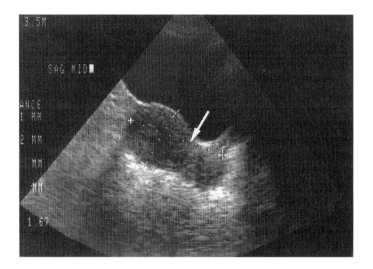

Use the above figure to answer question 3.116.

3.116 In this image, the arrow is MOST likely pointing to which part(s) of the uterus?
  A. fundus
  B. corpus
  C. isthmus
  D. cervix

C is correct.
The isthmus is the area where the corpus becomes the cervix and is the most flexible part of the uterus, being where the uterus bends when the bladder is empty. The corpus or body of the uterus contains the main part of the uterine cavity and is located just below the fundus, the rounded area above the uterine cavity. The cornua of the uterus (parts of the fundus) are located at the points of attachment of the Fallopian tubes.

3.117 The age of the subject whose uterus measures 2.5 cm in length and has a cervix-to-fundus ratio of 2:1 is MOST likely _____ years.
  A. 6
  B. 14
  C. 24
  D. 64

A is correct.
The pediatric uterus starts growing under the influence of pubertal gonadotropins at ± 8 years of age, reaching 6 cm by ± 13 years. The cervix-to-corpus length ratio remains 2:1. With puberty and adulthood, the uterus achieves its normal non-parous length of 9–10 cm with a cervix-to-corpus length ratio of 1:2. After menopause, the uterus undergoes atrophy and technically returns to a smaller size, with a cervix-to-corpus length ratio of 2:1. However, due to factors such as previous parity or fibroids, the ultimate size and shape of the postmenopausal uterus may vary from 6–10 cm; the cervix may be slightly more prominent than the fundus. These changes reflect alterations in the muscular layer of the corpus. The cervix varies least in size with age.

3.118 The part of the uterine wall that is NOT sonographically distinct is the:
   A. endometrium
   B. myometrium
   C. serosa
   D. all are sonographically distinct

C is correct.

The outer serosal layer is very thin and not sonographically visible. It is continuous with the pelvic fascia. The myometrium is composed of three layers of muscle fibers interwoven with loose connective tissue, blood and lymph vessels, and nerves. The muscle layers of the cervix contain more elastin and collagen than are found in the myometrium. The endometrial layer, or mucosa, is sonographically distinct, and contains connective and glandular tissue. It is continuous with the vaginal lining and the peritoneum through the tubal lining. Its appearance varies with the phase of the menstrual cycle as well as with pregnancy, infection, tumor, IUDs, etc.

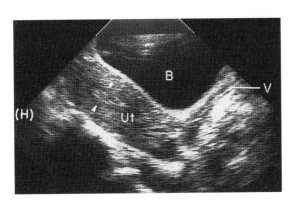

Use the above figure to answer question 3.119.

3.119 This image of the endometrium is MOST compatible with which of the following phases of the menstrual cycle?
   A. menstrual
   B. postmenstrual
   C. proliferative
   D. secretory

D is correct.

Normal endometrial thickness is greatest just prior to menstruation (secretory phase) and should not exceed 12–14 mm. During the secretory phase, the endometrium is highly echogenic. The subsequent menstrual endometrium is a thin echogenic line. At 3–4 days postmenstruation, the endometrium appears anechoic and measures 2–4 mm; it gradually builds up to a slightly echogenic proliferative endometrium of ± 4–8 mm to the secretory phase. During the proliferative phase, a hypoechoic layer can be seen within the more echogenic layers of endometrium which may represent edema. Endometrial measurement should not include the outer hypoechoic layer, which is myometrial in origin and probably contains extensive vascular structures.

3.120 Uterine cervical length in nulliparous women is MOST usually _____.
  A. 1–2 cm
  B. 2–3 cm
  C. 3–4 cm
  D. 4–5 cm

B is correct.
The full bladder required for a transabdominal sonogram, however, may cause the cervix to appear longer than it really is. If a cervix during pregnancy appears < 3 cm, it may be indicative of cervical incompetence.

3.121 Which of the following structures is MOST likely to contain mucosa which impedes the migration of bacteria?
  A. vagina
  B. cervix
  C. corpus
  D. fundus

B is correct.
The endothelium of the cervix is distinctive in that its mucosa is arranged in folds that slant downwards towards the external os. The mucus impedes the upward movement of bacteria. In addition, the endometrium of the corpus contains cilia, which propel mucus towards the cervix. Thus, the endometrium and endocervical canal are normally bacteria-free. The amount of endocervical mucus is usually greatest at the onset of pregnancy, when it forms a dense sticky mucus plug.

3.122 In comparison to the posterior wall of the vagina, the anterior wall is:
  A. longer
  B. shorter
  C. the same length
  D. wider

B is correct.
The inferior end of the cervix inserts into this oblique structure, forming a pocket (fornix) of the vaulted dead-end space between the inner vaginal wall and outer surface of the lower cervix. The vagina is thin-walled, ± 7–10 cm in length and very flexible.

3.123 The inner lining of the vagina is composed of:
  A. stratified squamous epithelium
  B. ciliated mucosa
  C. glandular endometrium
  D. a thin fibrous layer

A is correct.
The vaginal epithelium is **non-keratinized** stratified squamous epithelium and is continuous with the perineal surface. The endovaginal canal is usually collapsed into a flat H-shape, forming a potential space.

3.124 Which of the following structures is/are NOT covered by peritoneum?
  A. uterus
  B. Fallopian tubes
  C. ovaries
  D. urinary bladder

C and D are correct.
The peritoneum covers the uterine fundus and corpus, and is then reflected back, skirting the superior portion of the bladder and anterior portion of the distal colon to envelop the isthmus portion of the tubes. It forms the broad ligament at the lateral margins of the uterus. A portion of the posterior broad ligament extends outwards to form the mesovarium, which attaches at the hilus of the ovary and provides vascular access to that organ (along with the infundibulopelvic ligament). The ovarian ligament is a cord running within the broad ligament from the medial aspect of the ovary to the lateral portion of the uterus and inferior to the Fallopian tube. The ovarian germinal epithelium (outer layer) is continuous with the mesovarium, but is sufficiently different so as not to be considered peritoneal tissue. The tunica albuginea is a thin layer of fibrous tissue lying immediately beneath the germinal epithelium.

3.125 The number of primordial follicles persisting to adult life and progressing to ovulation is MOST usually:
  A. 100–200
  B. 300–400
  C. 600–700
  D. > 1000

B is correct.
Only some of the follicles present at birth undergo maturational development and ovulation, and no new follicles are produced during the lifespan of the ovaries. Each ovary releases one egg every other month in turn. Of the thousands of primordial follicles contained in the cortex of the ovary (comprising the bulk of ovarian parenchyma), only 300–400 eventually mature.

3.126 The mature follicle which ruptures at ovulation is called a:
  A. preantral follicle
  B. Graafian follicle
  C. corpus luteum
  D. corpus albicans

B is correct.
The medulla in the center of the ovary contains blood vessels and connective tissue. A developing preantral follicle migrates from the cortex towards the outer germinal epithelium, becoming a mature Graafian follicle (1.5–2.0 cm). With ovulation, the follicle ruptures and the egg is released. The follicle remnant then develops into a thick-walled blood-filled corpus luteum which, if no fertilization occurs, involutes into a corpus albicans. If fertilization does take place, the corpus luteum enlarges and becomes a corpus luteum of pregnancy, which produces the hormones necessary to sustain the developing placenta. This, too, involutes after the second month of pregnancy, when the placenta becomes stabilized.

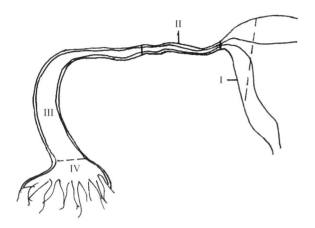

Use the above figure to answer question 3.127.

3.127 In this image, the portion of the Fallopian tube designated as 'III' is the:
  A. ampulla
  B. interstitium
  C. isthmus
  D. fimbriated infundibulum

A is correct.
The ampulla and infundibulum are not enclosed in the broad ligament. The broad ligament at this point forms the infundibulopelvic ligament, which attaches the posterior portion of this part of the tube to the lateral pelvic wall. A lateral portion of the mesovarium provides attachment for one of the fimbriae to the lateral portion of the ovary. The tubes are composed of an outer serosal layer (continuous with overlying peritoneum only at the isthmic portion), a muscular layer and a mucosa, which is continuous with uterine endometrium.

3.128 In which of the following areas is fertilization MOST likely to take place?
  A. germinal endothelium of the ovary
  B. abdominal cavity
  C. fimbriated infundibulum
  D. ampulla

D is correct.
Only in rare instances does fertilization take place elsewhere. The fertilized ovum is propelled through the tube by muscular contractions of the tube. It takes around 3–4 days for the fertilized ovum to pass through the oviduct (tube). During this passage, the fertilized ovum develops through a morula stage (solid mass of cells) to become a blastocyst, in which a single layer of cells (primitive trophoblast) surrounds a semifluid-filled cavity with an inner cell mass of rapidly dividing cells (embryonic pole and primitive endoderm) at one pole. This blastocyst implants in the uterine lining 7–8 days after ovulation.

3.129 The cervix is anchored so that its axis is generally parallel to the central body axis by the:
A. round ligament
B. broad ligament
C. cardinal ligament
D. uterosacral ligament

D is correct.
The cardinal ligaments (transverse cervical ligaments) are ill-defined bands of fibro-muscular tissue originating from the lateral aspect of the cervix and uterine corpus. They insert over a large area of the lateral pelvic wall and posteriorly to the sacrum. The posterior bands are more condensed and form the uterosacral ligaments.

3.130 The fibromuscular bands which originate from the uterine cornua and extend anteriorly across the pelvic brim are the:
A. round ligaments
B. broad ligaments
C. infundibulopelvic ligaments
D. ovarian ligaments

A is correct.
After passing through the pelvic brim, they extend through the inguinal ring and become anchored in the external genitalia.

3.131 Reflection of the peritoneum from the posterior wall of the uterus to the posterior pelvic wall, covering the rectum, forms the:
A. pouch of Douglas
B. vesicouterine pouch
C. posterior cul-de-sac
D. rectouterine pouch

A, C and D are correct.
These are all names for the same potential space, which forms the most posterior and inferior portion of the peritoneum lining the abdominopelvic cavity. This space extends downwards posterior to the cervix and up to the uterosacral ligaments. The vesicouterine pouch is the potential space formed by the reflection of peritoneum from the anterior wall of the uterus and posterior urinary bladder.

3.132 The most anterior and lateral of the three tubular structures seen on a sagittal view of the pelvis lateral to the uterus at the level of the ovary is the:
A. hypogastric artery
B. external iliac artery
C. internal iliac vein
D. ureter

D is correct.
The internal iliac artery (hypogastric artery) courses posterior and slightly medial to the ureter, with the internal iliac vein being the most posterior vessel. These are all visualized sonographically superolateral to the ovary, with the ureter coursing posterior to the ovary as it approaches the bladder.

3.133 The left ovarian vein drains into which of the following?
A. IVC
B. left renal vein
C. umbilical vein
D. internal iliac vein

B is correct.
The embryonic ovaries originate in the abdomen from the same mesenchyme as do the adrenal glands. They descend into the pelvis, bringing their main vascular supply with them (although blood is also brought to the ovaries by the adnexal branch of the hypogastric artery). Thus, although the uterus is supplied by branches of the internal iliac artery, the main arterial supply of the ovaries originates higher up in the aorta, just inferior to the renal vessels. The ovarian veins follow the course of the arteries, with the right ovarian vein draining directly into the IVC. However, due to the location of the IVC to the right, it is more direct for the left ovarian vein to drain into the left renal vein.

Pelvic doppler

3.134 Doppler evaluation of an ovarian mass is MOST likely to show a(n):
   A. low pulsatility index
   B. high resistance flow
   C. increased diastolic flow
   D. lack of flow

A and C are correct.

Increased vascularization (neovascularity) is required for an ovarian mass to grow beyond 0.3–0.5 cm. Because these new vascular channels lack a muscular media, the resulting sinusoid spaces produce a low-impedance (low-resistance) flow. This is demonstrated on the Doppler spectral waveform by a high diastolic flow, reflecting a low pulsatility index. Low diastolic flow with high systolic flow is evidence of increased resistance, reflecting a high pulsatility index.

3.135 Ovarian torsion is MOST likely to produce which Doppler profile(s)?
   A. low pulsatility index
   B. high resistance flow
   C. increased diastolic flow
   D. lack of flow

B and D are correct.

With partial torsion, there is a high-resistance flow with absent or even reversed diastolic flow. With complete torsion, there is a complete lack of parenchymal blood flow.

Gynecologically related pathology

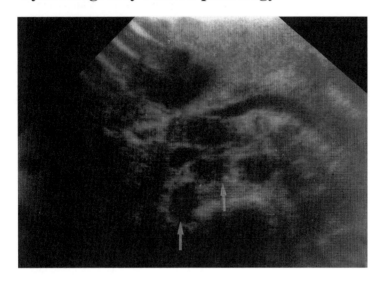

Use the above figure to answer question 3.136.

3.136 In this image, the arrows are MOST likely pointing to which structure(s)?

    A. lymphadenopathy
    B. endometrioma
    C. normal anatomy
    D. bowel tumor

A is correct.
Lymphadenopathy is often found in later stages of ovarian or, as in this case, cervical cancer. It is typically seen only when very enlarged. Groups of these lymph nodes appear as lobulated hypoechoic solid masses in the iliac or para-aortic region (as seen here). Endometriomas usually implant on the ligaments, and serosal surfaces of the bowel and peritoneum, and are very small and difficult to visualize sonographically. They may also cause renal obstruction if they implant near the ureters. Rupture of an intraperitoneal endometrioma containing clotted blood may result in acute peritonitis. A bowel mass can be recognized by its echogenic center, the bowel lumen.

3.137 An anechoic mass seen along the lateral vaginal wall is MOST probably a:

    A. bladder diverticulum
    B. hydroureter
    C. ureterocele
    D. Gartner's duct cyst

D is correct.
A Gartner's duct cyst is the result of incomplete obliteration of the atrophic mesonephric (Wolffian) duct in women. This duct remnant lies along the lateral vaginal wall. The cyst may be asymptomatic or may cause pain and swelling. The trigone area of the bladder (where the ureters enter) is located more medially and, therefore, a hydroureter at that point appears to be more anterior in relation to the vagina. A ureterocele is visualized within the urinary bladder at the trigone area. It is usually possible to visualize the connection between a bladder diverticulum and the bladder. Also, a diverticulum usually disappears on voiding.

3.138 Which of the following condition(s) is/are MOST often associated with pregancy?
  A. bladder diverticulum
  B. hydronephrosis
  C. gallstones
  D. pancreatic pseudocyst

B and C are correct.
The incidence of right-sided hydronephrosis appears to be higher than that on the left during pregnancy. Pressure exerted on the ureter by the gravid uterus is thought to be one cause of the ureteral and pelvic dilatation. Also, the high levels of progesterone during pregnancy may produce relaxation of the smooth muscles of the ureteral walls to accommodate the accompanying increase in pressure. Pregnancy may be a cause of gallbladder disease, possibly due to the increased gallbladder volume during pregnancy or to the associated decrease in concentration of bile salts and increase in cholesterol.

3.139 In the case of a hypoechoic lesion with irregular or poorly defined borders seen to the right of the uterus and in the cul-de-sac, what is/are the MOST likely differential diagnosis(es)?
  A. appendiceal abscess
  B. tuboovarian abscess
  C. twisted ovarian cyst
  D. normal colon

A, B and C are correct.
Any of these may be seen with these characteristics on sonography. Further evaluation is indicated. If there is doubt as to whether the mass represents normal colon, ultrasound monitoring after a water enema is the appropriate procedure.

Physiology

3.140 Ovarian follicular maturation beyond the preantral stage begins at:
  A. puberty
  B. birth
  C. release of gonadotropin releasing hormone (Gn-RH) from the hypothalamus
  D. corpus luteum formation

A and C are correct.
The thousands of primitive follicles present at birth represent oocytes arrested in the prophase of the ovulatory cycle. These either degenerate or continue on to maturation. Throughout childhood, follicular growth continues in some follicles to the next (preantral) stage, where they remain until puberty. At the onset of puberty, release of Gn-RH from the hypothalamus initiates cyclic and repetitive follicular development beyond the preantral stage. This follicular maturation continues throughout the reproductive period of life.

3.141 Oogenesis requires the cyclic influence of follicle-stimulating hormone (FSH) and luteinizing hormone (LH) produced by which structure(s)?
  A. hypothalamus
  B. anterior pituitary gland (adenohypophysis)
  C. posterior pituitary gland (neurohypophysis)
  D. adrenal gland

B is correct.
The production of FSH and LH in the anterior pituitary gland is in response to the influence of Gn-RH from the hypothalamus. FSH initiates follicular growth and maturation. The mature Graafian follicle secretes large amounts of estrogen into the circulation to trigger the release of LH. The LH surge causes ovulation/ follicular rupture, resulting in corpus luteum formation. The corpus luteum secretes estrogen and progesterone. As the effect of LH declines, the corpus luteum regresses, estrogen and progesterone production decreases, and endometrial shedding begins.

3.142 The dominant follicle that continues on to maturation is MOST likely to be sonographically detected endovaginally by day _____ of the menstrual cycle.
   A. 4
   B. 6
   C. 8
   D. 10

C is correct.
Of the six to eight preantral follicles that enlarge at the start of the menstrual cycle, usually only one becomes dominant and mature. At ± day 8, it measures 1.0 cm. The others undergo atresia. A follicle > 1.1 cm is a dominant follicle and matures to ovulation. At ovulation, the mean diameter is 2.0–2.4 cm.

3.143 The corpus luteum (or luteal) phase of the ovarian cycle lasts approximately _____ days.
   A. 6
   B. 10
   C. 14
   D. 18

C is correct.
After 14 days, the corpus luteum degenerates into a corpus albicans. However, if fertilization occurs, hCG is produced by the ovum, preventing corpus luteum regression. The corpus luteum of pregnancy then continues to produce estrogen and progesterone to further build up the endometrial lining of the uterus in preparation for implantation of the blastocyst. This continues until the placenta is established at around week 10 of gestation.

3.144 The endometrial layer that contains blood vessels and is NOT sloughed off during menstruation is the:
   A. functionalis
   B. compactum
   C. spongiosum
   D. basalis

D is correct.
The compactum and spongiosum together form the functionalis layer, that portion of endometrium which thickens and is shed at each menses. The basalis layer contains the nutrient vessels and remains intact. The proliferative and secretory phases of the endometrium coincide with the mid-to-late follicular phase and luteal phase of the ovulatory cycle, respectively.

3.145 An intrauterine gestational sac may be sono-graphically detected (endovaginally) by _____weeks.
   A. 2
   B. 4
   C. 6
   D. 8

B is correct.
This correlates with an hCG range of 1025 milliunits/ml (I.U., IRP) or 300–750 milliunits/ml (I.U., Second I.S.). The normal gestational sac can be visualized transabdominally by ± 6 weeks LMP. The embryonic pole can be seen by week 7.

3.146 In a patient with hCG levels < 1800 milliunits/ml (I.U., Second I.S.) and no sonographic evidence of an intrauterine gestational sac, what is/are the possible diagnosis(es)?
   A. intrauterine pregnancy
   B. ectopic pregnancy
   C. spontaneous abortion
   D. trophoblastic disease

A, B and C are correct.
It is possible that the low levels of hCG are simply indicative of very early pregnancy and, thus, no sac can be seen. As a rule, abnormal pregnancies, such as ectopics, produce low levels of hCG relative to sac size and also show a below-normal increase in hCG over 48 hours. Recent spontaneous abortions may also show evidence of low levels of hCG, but this becomes less evident if tested serially. Thus, low levels of hCG, with or without visualization of a gestational sac, cannot rule out ectopics. Trophoblastic disease, in contrast, tends to produce higher levels of hCG.

3.147 Fertilization is MOST likely to occur:
    A. imediately after ovulation
    B. 6–12 hours after ovulation
    C. 12–24 hours after ovulation
    D. 24–36 hours after ovulation

D is correct.
Fertilization usually occurs in the ampullary portion of the tube. The sperm penetrates the outer layer of the ovum, the zona pellucida. The tail of the sperm remains outside the ovum while the genetic material in the head of the sperm and the nucleus of the ovum merge to form a single cell, the zygote. Mitosis (cell division) begins within a few hours and the developing zygote (morula) is propelled though the tube. When the zygote reaches the uterus, the zona pellucida disappears and the developing blastocyst begins to receive nutrients from the endometrial glands, although implantation has not yet occurred.

Pediatric

3.148 Precocious puberty is usually defined as the onset of the normal physiologic processes of puberty in girls before the age of _____ years.
    A. 4
    B. 6
    C. 8
    D. 10

C is correct.
In precocious puberty, the sequence of breast development, pubic and axillary hair development, and the onset of menstruation occur as is normally expected at puberty. The uterus and ovaries attain their postpubertal size and configuration. True precocious puberty, in contrast to the separate premature development of one or other pubertal characteristics, may be due to a lesion affecting the hypothalamus, but is usually idiopathic. Pseudo- or incomplete precocious puberty may be due to one of several adrenal or ovarian dysfunctional processes, such as a granulosa-theca cell tumor or adrenal carcinoma.

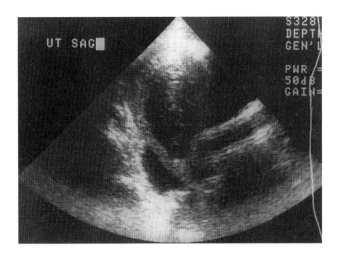

Use the above figure to answer question 3.149.

3.149 This image MOST probably represents:
   A. pyocolpos
   B. hydrometra
   C. pyometrocolpos
   D. hydrosalpinx

C is correct.
Pyometrocolpos is pus in the uterine endo-metrial canal and vagina. The others are, respectively, pus in the vagina, fluid in the uterus, and fluid in the tubes. If blood is present in these structures, the correct prefix is 'hemato'. The probable presence of pus and gas-forming organisms is indicated by the ring-down artifact in the fundus. Hydrometrocolpos makes up 15% of abdominal masses in infant girls. They are usually secondary to imperforate hymen, duplication anomaly with unilateral obstruction, or an acquired obstruction.

3.150 When a child with hydrocolpos does NOT have an imperforate hymen, the _____ should be evaluated.
   A. kidneys
   B. skeleton
   C. heart
   D. small intestine

A, B and C are correct.
There is a very high incidence of genital anomalies in females with renal anomalies. Skeletal and cardiac anomalies often accompany these conditions. Imperforate anus may also accompany hydrocolpos.

3.151 In a neonate, the presence of vaginal atresia, clitoromegaly, fused labia or cryptorchidism is MOST likely to indicate which of the following?
   A. Turner's syndrome
   B. dysgerminoma
   C. Meckel's syndrome
   D. ambiguous genitalia

D is correct.
In the presence of any of these findings, an effort should be made to locate the normal uterus, vagina, ovaries and/or testes, as well as evaluate the kidneys and adrenals. The various conditions of ambiguous genitalia or hermaphroditism may be due to congenital adrenal hyperplasia, increased/decreased androgen production or an enzyme defect.

3.152 The ovaries in a pediatric patient normally measure:
A. 1.5 × 0.25 × 0.3 cm
B. 1.5 × 0.25 × 0.3 mm
C. 3 × 2 × 2 cm
D. 3 × 2 × 2 mm

A is correct.
At birth, the ovaries have usually descended to their normal location in the pelvis. Before puberty, ovarian volume is 1 cm^3, which increases to ± 6 cm^3 in adulthood.

3.153 A cystic mass in the ovary of a child is MOST likely to represent a:
A. benign cystic teratoma
B. serous cystadenoma of childhood
C. vesicouterine reflux through the Fallopian tube
D. delayed regression of a premenarchal follicle

D is correct.
Pediatric ovarian cysts are usually not a cause for concern. Follicles in varying stages of development are always present; it is estimated that up to 5% of neonatal ovaries contain cysts > 0.7 cm in diameter. These cysts may be seen throughout childhood and usually involve follicles that do not contain ova.

Infertility

3.154 An intrauterine contraceptive device (IUD) functions by preventing:
A. ovulation
B. transport of sperm
C. fertilization
D. implantation in the uterus

D is correct.
Different IUDs work in different ways to prevent implantation. Some types release copper, causing the endometrial tissues to be premature and out of phase with ovulation. Others release progesterone, which slows endometrial development and changes the viscosity of the cervical mucus without changing the ovulatory cycle.

3.155 Which of the following is MOST likely to be associated with IUD use?
A. pregnancy
B. septic abortion
C. pelvic inflammatory disease (PID)
D. ectopic pregnancy

All are correct.
Even when the IUD is correctly placed, it is not 100% effective. If pregnancy occurs, the IUD is usually removed immediately. If this is not possible, the pregnancy must be closely monitored, as there may be an increased incidence of spontaneous abortion and sepsis. The string of the IUD is a potential route of infection, leading to a higher incidence of PID with IUD use. The risk of ectopic pregnancy with IUD use is reportedly 5–10 times higher than normal, and may remain so even after the IUD has been removed.

3.156 Which of the following is NOT considered a cause of infertility?
   A. pelvic inflammatory disease (PID)
   B. endometriosis
   C. congenital anomaly
   D. retroverted uterus
   E. varicocele

D is correct.
The version of the uterus has no effect on its function. Although a retroverted uterus may have ovaries located more eccentrically than with an anteverted uterus, there is no effect on function. Scarring and adhesions from PID, obstruction due to endometriosis (especially in the tubes), congenital anomalies and diethylstilbestrol (DES) exposure are all causes of infertility in women, and are unrelated to problems of ovulation. Varicoceles in the male scrotum lead to infertility due to the increase in temperature accompanying the increased blood flow around the testes.

3.157 The MOST likely ovulatory cause of infertility related to ovulation is:
   A. polycystic ovary disease (PCOD)
   B. hypogonadotropism
   C. stress
   D. pituitary tumor

A is correct.
In PCOD patients, the pituitary–ovarian feedback mechanism is acyclic. The ovaries secrete hormones in improper amounts, and oligomenorrhea or amenorrhea and anovulation are usually present. Hypogonadotropism (increased FSH and LH) is a condition characterized by anestrogenic amenorrhea with no follicles in the ovaries. These patients do not respond to ovarian stimulation. Pituitary tumors such as microadenomas may be the cause of hypogonadotropism. Removal of the tumor may bring about a return of normal ovulation. Although stress is a factor that may contribute to hormone imbalance, it is not directly causative.

3.158 Ovulation induction by hormone therapy is used to treat disorders caused by:
   A. endometriosis
   B. congenital anomalies
   C. obstruction
   D. dysfunction of pituitary–ovarian feedback system

D is correct.
Endometriosis and congenital anomalies can be either corrected or approached through a mechanical form of treatment. Obstructions such as adhesions are often the cause of ectopic pregnancies. Ovulation induction is used when lack of ovulation is observed, an indication that the pituitary–hypothalamic–ovarian axis is inadequate to stimulate follicular growth. Lack of ovulation is established by hormonal assay and basal body-temperature evaluation.

3.159 During the ovulatory cycle, a dominant follicle(s) appear(s) between _____ days.
   A. 1 and 4
   B. 5 and 8
   C. 8 and 12
   D. 15 and 20

C is correct.
The dominant follicle(s) is/are usually 14–18 mm in diameter and usually grow 2–3 mm/ day. Patients undergoing hormone-induction therapy receive Clomid™ or Pergonal® on day 1 and hCG when the follicle reaches 18 mm. The follicle(s) then grow to 20–24 mm, whereupon ovulation occurs (24–36 hours after hCG is administered).

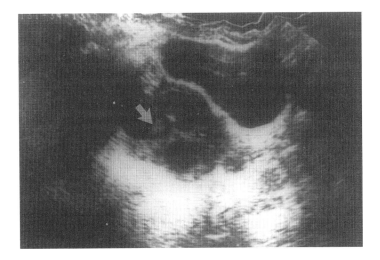

Use the above figure to answer question 3.160.

3.160 In this image, the structure within the ovarian follicle to which the arrow is MOST likely pointing is a:
    A. cumulus oophorus
    B. thickened follicular contour
    C. follicular carcinoma
    D. corpus luteum cyst

A is correct.
The cumulus oophorus is a sonographically detectable sign of impending ovulation, appearing as a small echogenic cone projecting into the follicle which represents granulosa cells surrounding the oocyte. It may be seen within 36 hours prior to ovulation.

3.161 Which of the following is MOST likely to be associated with theca-lutein cysts as a result of ovulation induction?
    A. multiple pregnancy
    B. ovarian hyperstimulation syndrome (OHSS)
    C. ectopic pregnancy
    D. endometrial hyperplasia

B is correct.
OHSS is a serious potential complication of ovulation induction. Development of multiple follicles and bilateral theca-lutein cysts cause the ovaries to become grossly enlarged, on occasions > 10 cm in diameter. Increased levels of hCG cause ovarian stromal edema and very high estrogen levels. Depending on the degree of severity, symptoms may include moderate-to-severe lower abdominal pain, ascites, pleural effusion and ruptured ovary. The symptoms either resolve or, if pregnancy occurs, linger for 6–8 weeks.

3.162 A predisposing condition encouraging the use of *in vitro* fertilization (IVF-ET) or gamete interfallopian transfer (GIFT) procedures is MOST likely to be:
    A. polycystic ovaries
    B. endometriosis
    C. dysfunctional pituitary–ovarian feedback system
    D. sperm inadequacy

B is correct.
Endometriosis may cause adhesions to block at least one of the tubes. With IVF, several mature follicles are retrieved under ultrasound guidance (after hormonal stimulation) The ova are then fertilized in a culture dish and the resulting embryo(s) transferred to the uterus for implantation (48–72 h after ova fertilization). The success rate is 10–25%. Ultrasound is performed before oocyte retrieval to ensure that premature ovulation has not occurred. If only one tube is blocked, the GIFT procedure is more appropriate. With this procedure, both the sperm and oocyte are inserted into the Fallopian tube for subsequent fertilization.

Postmenopause

3.163 Because the endometrium in postmenopausal women is atrophic, on sonography, the endometrial echo is MOST likely to measure around _____ in its anteroposterior dimension.
- A. 1–2 mm
- B. 2–4 mm
- C. 6–8 mm
- D. 10–12 mm

C is correct.
If the postmenopausal endometrium is > 1 cm, dilatation and curettage may be performed (especially if there is accompanying bleeding). Note, however, that the postmenopausal endometrium may be up to 1 cm thick if the patient has been undergoing estrogen-replacement therapy.

3.164 Ovarian function is MOST likely to decline in the fifth decade due to:
- A. fewer follicles
- B. decreasing estrogen
- C. decreasing androgen
- D. decreasing progesterone

A is correct.
The ovaries are less able to respond to pituitary gonadotropins (hypothalamic–pituitary–ovarian feedback system) because there are fewer viable follicles primarily because of follicular atresia. Therefore, the ovaries eventually secrete less estrogen, and ovulation and menstruation become irregular and ultimately cease.

3.165 If the endometrium in a postmenopausal woman is > 1.0 cm, which of the following is MOST likely to be contributory?
- A. endometrial hyperplasia
- B. endometrial polyps
- C. blood or mucus within the lumen
- D. endometrial carcinoma

All are correct.
Endometrial thickening may be due to endometrial hyperplasia, which may be the result of exogenous estrogen or an estrogen-producing tumor. In this age group, endometrial cancer should first be ruled out. Polyps may also be seen as endometrial thickening, but are more irregular and echogenic. Polyps rarely undergo malignant change; however, in the postmenopausal woman, as polyps may arise in an area of hyperplasia, endometrial carcinoma should be considered.

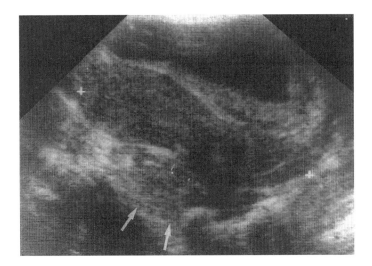

Use the above figure to answer question 3.166.

3.166 In this image, which is the MOST likely condition being visualized?

    A. endometrial carcinoma
    B. carcinoma of the cervix
    C. adenomyosis
    D. leiomyoma

B is correct.

The incidence of carcinoma of the cervix is approximately half that of endometrial carcinoma, most probably because of the increasing use of the Papanicolaou test for cervical cancer. Risk factors include early sexual activity, multiple sex partners and herpesvirus type 2 infection. In the case shown here, a stage IV cancer has spread to the bladder wall and posterior cul-de-sac.

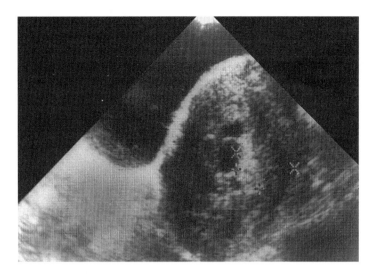

Use the above figure to answer question 3.167.

3.167 In this image of the uterus of a 79-year-old patient with a history of postmenopausal bleeding, what is/are the MOST likely diagnosis(es)?
   A. endometrial carcinoma
   B. carcinoma of the cervix
   C. adenomyosis
   D. leiomyoma

A is correct.

The irregular thickening of the endometrium and fluid collections in the endometrial cavity most likely represent blood and tissue necrosis. There is probably myometrial extension of the tumor. Endometrial carcinoma is a disease primarily of postmenopausal women; it also has a high correlation with obesity, diabetes and hypertension in older women. Around one-third of patients with postmenopausal bleeding have endometrial carcinoma. The ultrasound appearance is variable and non-specific, but the more highly differentiated tumors with mucin and glandular elements tend to be more echogenic than other types. There is mounting evidence that color-flow Doppler may be helpful in distinguishing altered flow patterns and low pulsatility indices due to neovascularization.

3.168 In multiparous women aged 40–50 years, the MOST likely benign cervical neoplasm to occur is:
   A. cervical myoma
   B. Gartner's duct cyst
   C. adenomyosis
   D. cervical polyp

D is correct.

Remember that cysts are not neoplasms. Cervical polyps rarely occur in postmenopausal women. They are usually attached to the cervical wall by pedicles and may grow to several centimeters in size. They are usually seen as small echogenic foci. Adenomyosis, a benign condition in which endometrial tissue grows in the myometrium, is seen in women > 50 years of age. Symptoms are dysmenorrhea and abnormal bleeding, which may be secondary to increased estrogen levels. Adenomyosis may be either focal or diffuse, leading to an enlarged uterus. It may be seen in association with leiomyomas and may be mistaken for endometriosis.

Pelvic pathology

3.169 A cystic pelvic mass encountered in a postmenopausal woman is MOST likely to be:

A. a physiologic ovarian cyst
B. polycystic ovarian disease
C. cystadenoma
D. fibroma

C is correct.
The first two are conditions encountered in women of reproductive age. Cystadenomas, the most common type of ovarian tumors, may become rather large, with septations and/or papillary protrusions. They are generally benign. The presence of solid and irregular-looking tissue within a cystic structure is an indication of possible malignancy. Fibromas are solid ovarian masses. Both may be associated with ascites.

3.170 Which of the following epidemiological factors is/are MOST likely to predispose to ovarian carcinoma?

A. increased number of years of ovulatory activity
B. early menopause
C. family history of ovarian cancer
D. family history of breast cancer

A, C and D are correct.
A direct relationship has been shown between the risk of developing ovarian carcinoma and the number of years of ovulation. It is thought that incessant and prolonged years of ovulation may cause minor trauma to the surface epithelium of the ovary, which may prepare the way for ovarian carcinoma. Also, certain environmental factors have been linked to the development of ovarian cancer. Japan appears to be the only industrialized country with a low risk of this disease. The peak incidence of ovarian cancer is at ages 55–59 years.

3.171 If a congenital uterine anomaly is found, which system(s) should the sonographer examine for possible related anomalies?

A. gastrointestinal
B. cardiac
C. skeletal
D. urinary

D is correct.
Although congenital uterine anomalies are uncommon overall, they are seen in approximately 50% of patients with such congenital urinary tract disorders as absence of one kidney. Congenital uterine anomalies associated with pregnancy may lead to complications such as spontaneous abortion, PROM and abnormal fetal positions.

3.172 Visualization of an intrauterine pregnancy together with an empty endometrial stripe is MOST likely to indicate the presence of:

A. uterus arcuatus
B. uterus subseptus
C. uterus bicornis
D. uterus didelphys

B, C and D are correct.
These are various degrees of uterine septation/ duplication, from the least (arcuatus), which is an indentation in the fundal wall, to the most (didelphys), in which the septation extends the length of the uterus. In early pregnancy, depending on the plane used to scan the non-gravid portion of the uterus, the endometrium of the contralateral horn of the uterus – without the gestational sac – may be seen. The endometrium is thickened due to hormonal stimulation (decidual reaction), but the double rind of pregnancy is absent. As the pregnancy grows in size, the duplicated portion of the uterus becomes no longer visible.

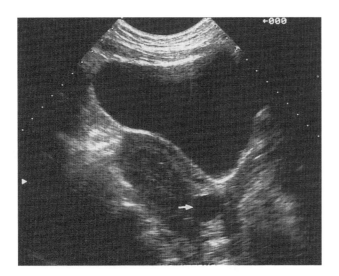

Use the above figure to answer question 3.173.

3.173 In this image, the arrow is MOST likely pointing to a:

    A. Gartner's duct cyst

    B. Morgagni cyst

    C. parovarian cyst

    D. Nabothian cyst

D is correct.

Nabothian cysts are typically small retention cysts of the cervix seen within the endocervical canal. Cysts of Morgagni, a type of parovarian cyst, arise from the fimbriated end of the tube and appear as adnexal masses. All parovarian cysts arise in the mesovarium from Wolffian duct remnants and appear as adnexal masses. They are usually small, but may become quite large and may twist or become hemorrhagic. Gartner's duct cysts are found in the lateral vaginal wall.

3.174 The MOST common cause(s) of disruption of the uterine contour in a woman at any age is/are:

    A. endometriosis

    B. leiomyoma

    C. adenomyosis

    D. polyps

B is correct.

Around 20–25% of women > 35 years of age are estimated to have leiomyomas (fibroids). The occurrence is greater in black women. Myomas may be found in the cervix and even in the broad ligament but, most usually, they are found in the corpus of the uterus. Description is according to their location. Subserous myomas lie under the peritoneal (serosal) surface of the uterus and may become pedunculated. Intramural myomas lie within the myometrium, and submucous myomas develop under the endometrium and often cause distortion of the endometrial cavity.

3.175 A solid mass found during pregnancy is MOST likely to be:
   A. endometriosis
   B. leiomyoma
   C. adenomyosis
   D. polyps

B is correct.

Due to the effect of increases in estrogen during pregnancy, myomas may increase in size, although most do not. There is usually no effect on the pregnancy unless the size or location of the myoma impinges on the fetus or the cervix. Myomas at or near the cervix may prevent vaginal delivery; those near the placenta place it at risk of premature rupture of membranes, antepartum bleeding and post-partum hemorrhage. It is important to differentiate a myoma from a uterine contraction. Fibroid echogenicity is usually less than that of myometrium or the placenta. Also, myomas are well circumscribed, attenuate sound and occupy only a portion of the uterus.

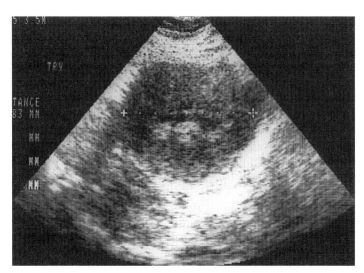

Use the above figure to answer question 3.176.

3.176 In this image, what is/are the MOST likely condition(s) represented?
   A. endometriosis
   B. leiomyoma
   C. adenomyosis
   D. polyps

D is correct.

Endometrial polyps may appear as focal echogenicities, as seen here, or they may appear as thickening of the central endometrial echo. Abnormal endometrial echogenicity and thickening (> 10 mm) should prompt further evaluation. Differential diagnoses for this finding include endometrial hyperplasia and carcinoma.

3.177 The MOST likely location(s) of a pedunculated leiomyoma is/are:
- A. the cervical area
- B. the lower uterine segment
- C. lateral to the uterine fundus
- D. superior to the uterine fundus

D is correct.

These are subserosal myomas which have grown out of the uterine corpus. They may even extend past the broad ligament and may be mistaken for an extrauterine mass. The pedunculated myoma exhibits the typical heterogeneous appearance of a myoma. As pedunculated myomas are attached by a thin pedicle, they often lose their blood supply and become necrotic, and appear to be entirely or partially anechoic. It is important to differentiate a pedunculated myoma from a solid ovarian mass. If it is indeed a myoma, the normal ovary is then seen as distinct from the mass, and other myomas are likely to be found in the uterus.

3.178 Acute enlargement of a cystic ovarian mass is MOST likely to be caused by:
- A. metastatic spread
- B. internal hemorrhage
- C. venous engorgement
- D. tubal obstruction

B and C are correct.

Venous engorgement is most likely to occur secondary to adnexal torsion. In such cases, echoes may be seen inside the cystic structure representing cellular debris, pus, organized blood or sebaceous material.

3.179 Hydrosalpinx is MOST likely to be caused by:
- A. metastatic spread
- B. internal hemorrhage
- C. venous engorgement
- D. tubal obstruction

D is correct.

The Fallopian tube is not normally visualized sonographically unless pathology is present. A common cause of tubal obstruction is adhesions secondary to inflammation, as in salpingitis. Because of the obstruction (which may also be due to iatrogenic ligation, endometriosis and tumor), intraluminal secretions may become trapped within the tube, causing dilation. The resulting anechoic tubal structure seen on ultrasound is usually narrower where it enters the uterine cornu. It may be differentiated from fluid-filled bowel by the lack of peristalsis. If the ovary is involved in the inflammatory process, it is called a tuboovarian abscess, which generally has a more complex sonographic appearance.

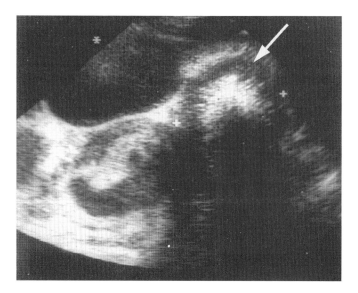

Use the above figure to answer question 3.180.

3.180 In this transverse view of the pelvis, the structure indicated by the arrow is MOST likely to be a:
    A. cystadenoma
    B. dermoid/benign cystic teratoma
    C. dysgerminoma
    D. left adnexal ectopic pregnancy

B is correct.
Dermoid cysts are the most common type of germ cell tumor. They are generally seen in women of childbearing age. These cysts may contain varying types of tissue, such as fat, skin, teeth and hair. On sonography, they appear as a complex, mostly solid, mass with echogenic components or, as seen here, as a mostly echogenic rounded mass with fluid anteriorly and posterior shadowing. The posterior shadowing is important for the diagnosis as few other adnexal masses exhibit acoustic shadowing. They may also appear cystic or contain a fluid-fluid level. Dysgerminomas and endodermal sinus tumors are less common malignant types of germ cell tumors.

3.181 Cystic ovarian masses are often septate. When the walls or septations are thickened (> 0.3 mm), this is MOST likely to be associated with:
    A. normal cystic degeneration
    B. inflammation
    C. endometriosis
    D. malignancy

B, C and D are correct.
In a sonographically complex adnexal mass, the presence of echogenic components indicates a greater risk of malignancy, although highly echogenic components may also be present in benign dermoid cysts. Other signs of malignancy are ascites and adherent bowel loops.

3.182 Simple adnexal cysts > 10.0 cm:
    A. usually regress spontaneously
    B. usually have thickened septa
    C. are usually corpus luteum cysts
    D. have a greater potential to become malignant

D is correct.
As these larger cysts seldom spontaneously regress and have a greater potential than smaller cysts of becoming malignant, they are usually removed. Although thickened septa indicate a greater risk of malignancy, many very large cystic masses are simple cysts with or without thin septa.

3.183 Which of the following is MOST likely to be relieved by the onset of menopause?
    A. endometriosis
    B. pelvic inflammatory disease
    C. cystadenoma
    D. Brenner tumor

A is correct.
Endometriosis is related to cyclic hormonal stimulation, which ceases after natural menopause or post-hysterectomy with bilateral oophorectomy. PID is an inflammatory condition unrelated to age, and cystadenomas and Brenner tumors are usually associated with older women.

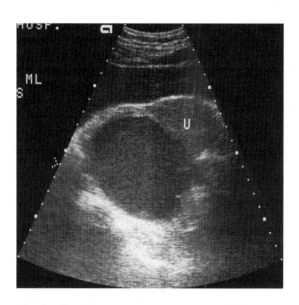

Use the above figure to answer question 3.184.

3.184 In this image, the mass is LEAST likely to be a(n):
    A. hemorrhagic ovarian cyst
    B. uterine fibroid
    C. endometrioma
    D. mucinous cystadenoma

B is correct.
Endometriosis may be focal or diffuse. Sonographic findings are variable and may range from cystic to solid to complex. The characteristic 'chocolate-cyst' appearance of an endometrioma filled with old blood is usually 2–5 cm in diameter, but may exceed 10 cm. Endometriosis is commonly found bilaterally in the ovaries, but may be seen in the cervix, vagina, posterior cul-de-sac or broad ligaments. Rarely, implantation occurs around areas of previous surgery, such as in the umbilicus, bladder and other parts of the body. Note that a hemorrhagic ovarian cyst may be indistinguishable from an endometrioma. Mucinous cystadenomas are often septated, but may also resemble this image.

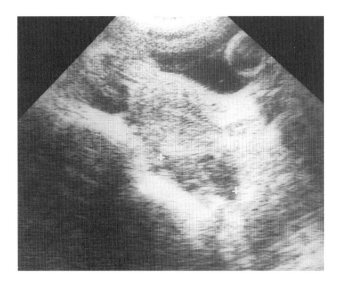

Use the above figure to answer question 3.185.

3.185 Which of the following conditions is/are MOST likely to be represented by this image?
  A. Stein–Leventhal syndrome
  B. Meckel's syndrome
  C. Crohn's disease
  D. Marfan syndrome

A is correct.
Stein–Leventhal syndrome, also known as polycystic ovary disease, is an endocrine disorder associated with obesity, oligomenorrhea, hirsutism and infertility. This disorder often produces bilaterally enlarged ovaries that contain multiple, poorly developed (2–6 mm), peripheral cysts. In many cases, the enlarged ovaries are visualized adjacent to and below the uterus in the cul-de-sac, leading to the term 'kissing ovaries'. In approximately 25–33% of symptomatic patients, the ovaries appear normal. In the presence of some of the clinical symptoms of PCOD, such as oligomenorrhea and infertility, but without the sonographic appearance, a form of adrenal tumor should also be considered. However, some patients with true PCOD as well as the characteristic sonographic appearance may present with no clinical symptoms whatsoever.

Pelvic Doppler

3.186 Bilaterally enlarged ovaries containing multiple small cysts are MOST likely to be seen in which of the following?
  A. female neonates
  B. polycystic ovary disease
  C. ovulation induction
  D. Brenner tumor

A, B and C are correct.
The sonographic appearance of PCOD may be seen in women receiving follicle-stimulating hormone therapy although, in such cases, the cysts are more likely to be larger, thicker-walled, theca-lutein cysts. The ovaries of female newborns may still be subject to stimulation by maternal hormones, producing a similar ovarian appearance. Brenner tumor presents as a solid adnexal mass in older women and is not to be confused with PCOD.

3.187 The use of Clomid to induce ovulation is MOST likely to cause which of the following Doppler findings?
    A. low pulsatility waveforms in both ovarian arteries
    B. high pulsatility waveforms in both ovarian arteries
    C. low pulsatility waveforms in one ovarian artery
    D. high pulsatility waveform in one ovarian artery

A is correct.
The administration of fertility drugs induces multiple follicle production in both ovaries, thereby producing a low-impedance (low-pulsatility) waveform.

3.188 Decreased perfusion in a uterine artery Doppler study is MOST likely to be caused by which of the following conditions?
    A. pelvic inflammatory disease (PID)
    B. ovulation induction
    C. severe endometriosis
    D. fibroids

A and C are correct.
This may be due to compromised vasodilation in the uterine artery as the result of scar tissue, or to the possible decrease in estradiol concentration in the uterine artery which may accompany PID and endometriosis. Vasodilation (leading to arterial perfusion) is affected by the level of estrogen present.

3.189 In Doppler studies of ovarian neoplasms, neovascularity is MOST likely to be seen in the presence of a(n):
    A. low pulsatility index
    B. high pulsatility index
    C. increased diastolic flow
    D. increased systolic flow

A and C are correct.
In ovarian neoplasms, neovascularity is required for growth to > 3–5 mm. The lack of muscular media in these masses leads to the development of sinusoid spaces around the periphery of the tumors. This produces a low-resistance system characterized by increased diastolic flow which translates to a low-pulsatility index. Low pulsatility is a non-specific finding that is seen in inflammatory masses, metabolically active tumors, germ cell tumors and corpus luteum cysts. The absence of a low-pulsatility index may rule out malignancy, as there is a high negative predictive value. However, because not all masses with low-pulsatility indices are malignant, the positive predictive value is lower.

Extrapelvic related pathology

3.190 Increased perfusion in the uterine artery is MOST likely to be seen in which of the following conditions?
    A. endometrial hyperplasia
    B. ovarian hyperstimulation syndrome
    C. pelvic inflammatory disease
    D. fibroids

A, B and D are correct.
These are all associated with increased estrogen levels, which is a contributory factor in increased perfusion. Therefore, an estrogen-secreting tumor also shows increased perfusion in the uterine artery.

3.191 The finding of > 10 ml of fluid in the cul-de-sac is MOST likely to be seen in which of the following conditions?
    A. benign ovarian mass
    B. malignant ovarian mass
    C. ovarian torsion
    D. normal finding

B and C are correct.
Although, on occasion, intraperitoneal fluid is seen with a benign adnexal mass, fluid is usually associated with malignant spread or rupture. With ovarian torsion, the fluid may represent exudate caused by the obstructed venous and lymphatic return. A small amount of fluid is normal in the cul-de-sac, but should not exceed 5–10 cc.

3.192 Which of the following is MOST likely to be involved in metastatic spread from a pelvic malignancy?

    A. heart

    B. kidneys

    C. lung

    D. liver

C and D are correct.

The liver is often a focus for metastases due to pelvic pathology, but carcinomas of the uterus and cervix have been shown to metastasize to the lung as well. Attention should also be paid to the para-aortic and paracaval areas as these may be involved by adenopathy. The kidneys are not likely to be involved in metastases, although a mass in the pelvis may obstruct one or both ureters, causing hydronephrosis. Thus, the kidneys should always be evaluated when a pelvic mass is present, regardless of whether or not it is malignant.

3.193 When a patient presents with an apparently normal kidney and an empty contralateral renal fossa, which of the following is/are the MOST likely differential diagnosis(es)?

    A. pelvic kidney

    B. duplicated urinary bladder

    C. uterus subseptus

    D. horseshoe kidney

A and C are correct.

If a kidney cannot be seen in the renal fossa and there is no evidence or history of the kidney having been removed, then the pelvic area should be carefully examined for a reniform structure. If not found, the uterus should also be carefully evaluated for septation or duplication, as renal agenesis is often seen in conjunction with uterine anomalies.

3.194 Rupture of a mucinous cystadenocarcinoma is MOST likely to cause which of the following?

    A. ascites

    B. meconium peritonitis

    C. fluid-filled endometrium

    D. pseudomyxoma peritonei

D is correct.

Pseudomyxoma peritonei is the condition characterized by intraperitoneal accumulation of a sticky gelatinous substance released by a ruptured or leaky mucinous cystadenocarcinoma (or a mucinous neoplasm of the appendix). Ascites is intraperitoneal fluid which is often seen with cirrhosis; it may also accompany many malignant, and some benign, neoplasms as well as some inflammatory conditions. Ascites is most often found in the cul-de-sac, left and right paracolic gutters, and Morrison's pouch. Malignant neoplasms may produce adhesions within the ascites. Both ascites and pseudomyxoma peritonei may lead to massive abdominal distention.

Patient care and technique

3.195 Which of the following neoplasms is MOST likely to present with metastases to the ovaries?

    A. endodermal sinus tumor

    B. Krukenberg's tumor

    C. neuroblastoma

    D. rhabdomyosarcoma

B, C and D are correct.

Endodermal sinus tumors are primary tumors of the ovaries. Krukenberg's tumors are primary to the gastrointestinal tract, and often metastasize to the ovaries in peri- and post-menopausal women. They commonly present as complex bilateral masses. Neuroblastomas often originate in the adrenal medulla of children and may occasionally metastasize to the ovaries. Rhabdomyoma and rhabdomyosarcoma are recurring neoplasms associated with tuberous sclerosis in children. They may be found anywhere in the body.

3.196 When an obstetric patient who has been bed-ridden for some time suddenly becomes dizzy or short of breath, the BEST action to take is to have the patient:

    A. raise her legs

    B. stand up and walk

    C. roll onto her right side

    D. roll onto her left side

D is correct.

These effects are the result of the supine position, which causes the weight of the fetus to press on the IVC, thereby preventing some of the blood from returning to the heart. The result is that less blood is sent into the systemic circulation. This situation is referred to as 'supine hypotensive syndrome' or 'caval compression syndrome'. Having the patient roll onto her left side alleviates the pressure on the IVC, allowing the return of normal blood flow. Elevating the patient's back may also prove helpful.

3.197 The MOST important biologic effect(s) of ultrasound is/are believed to be:

    A. thermal

    B. radiation

    C. pressure

    D. cavitation

A and D are correct.

A < 1° rise in temperature may occur during diagnostic ultrasound evaluation, but this has been experimentally shown to have no impact in humans. In the presence of stable gas-filled nuclei, cavitation may occur, but this is unlikely. In the 30 years that ultrasound has been used as a diagnostic tool, there have been "...no confirmed biological effects on patients or sonographers caused by exposure at intensities typical of present diagnostic ultrasound instruments." [AIUM Official Statement on Clinical Safety, approved October 1982; revised and approved March 1988] In a supporting statement in 1987, the AIUM declared, "In the low-megahertz frequency range, there have been no independently confirmed significant biological effects in mammalian tissues exposed *in vivo* to unfocused ultrasound with intensities below 100 mW/cm^2, or to focused ultrasound with intensities below 1 W/cm^2."

3.198 With a transvaginal probe, it is BEST to use a:
   A. probe cover if transmittable disease is suspected
   B. probe cover at all times
   C. disinfectant if transmittable disease is suspected
   D. disinfectant at all times

B and D are correct.

The microorganisms that cause sexually transmitted diseases may be transferred via the ultrasound probe. Therefore, a probe cover should be used at all times, and the examiner should always wear gloves. Condoms may be used instead of commercially available probe covers, but it should be remembered that these are thinner than probe covers and may break. Also, some condoms contain a spermicidal material which should not be used with infertility patients. The probe should be disinfected for 10 min after each use. Note that some disinfectants should not be used on some transducers, so attention should be paid to manufacturers' instructions.

3.199 To further assess a sonographically equivocal pelvic mass, it is BEST to have the patient:
   A. drink four glasses of water
   B. roll onto her left side
   C. take a water enema
   D. empty her bladder

C is correct.

In general, demonstrating peristalsis **around** a mass indicates that the mass is separate from the gastrointestinal system. However, peristalsis is not always seen, and the mass in question may represent normal bowel or a bowel mass. Ultrasound examination after adminis-tration of an enema allows documentation of the absence of the previously seen mass, or may improve visualization, thereby allowing determination of whether the mass is gynecologic or gastrointestinal in origin. If a mass is confirmed, the sonographer would be well advised to examine the kidneys for the presence of calyceal dilatation due to obstruction. In addition, there is always the chance that an unknown pelvic mass is a pelvic kidney; thus, examination of both renal fossae is recommended.

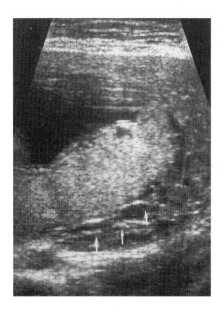

Use the above figure to answer question 3.200.

3.200 In this image, the arrow is MOST likely indicating which of the following?
    A. lifting of the placenta due to abruption
    B. normal maternal draining veins
    C. a subplacental uterine fibroid
    D. subplacental contraction

B is correct.
This is the normal hypoechoic appearance of normal maternal draining veins in the decidua basalis and myometrium. It is important not to confuse this with placental abruption or other pathology. Doppler interrogation of the area usually confirms its venous nature. The gravid uterus may also often present with prominent venous structures peripherally.

3.201 A simple cystic structure in the pelvis may appear sonographically complex MOST likely because of:
    A. slice thickness
    B. side lobe artifact
    C. enhancement
    D. attenuation

A and B are correct.
Side lobe artifacts are produced when multiple side beams of lower intensity than the main beam emerge from the transducer. These lower-intensity beams scatter the main beam against specular reflectors, such as the bladder, or diffuse reflectors, such as bowel gas, resulting in what appears to be debris in the urinary bladder. Slice thickness artifact is due to a 'partial volume' effect, as the sound beam has a certain width and diverges beyond the focal zone. The returning echoes are averaged with echoes from nearby interfaces. If a beam is adjacent to a cyst, the averaging effect of the cyst and surrounding tissue causes the cyst to appear echo-filled.

3.202 A sonographically visible mass not seen on a radiograph is termed a 'pseudomass'. This appearance is MOST likely to be due to:

    A. edge shadowing
    B. reverberation
    C. refraction
    D. attenuation

B is correct.

Reverberation, or multiple reflections of sound, occurs when the sound beam hits an interface with a large acoustic mismatch, such as soft tissue with gas or bone. When this happens, most of the sound is reflected back to the transducer and then re-reflected off the transducer back into the body. Thus, there is more than one reflection from the same interface, and each reflection is shown on the monitor. The greater the acoustic mismatch at the interface, the greater the number of reverberation echoes produced. When a highly reflective surface, such as the bladder, creates strong reverberation echoes, and when these echoes are superimposed on an anechoic or hypoechoic area, the false appearance of a mass is the result.